POCKET
NOTEBOOK

D0713591

Pocket
CARDIOLOGY

A Companion to Pocket Medicine

Editor

MARC S. SABATINE, MD, MPH

Authors

MARC P. BONACA, MD, MPH

GREGORY D. LEWIS, MD

MICHELLE L. O'DONOGHUE, MD, MPH

USHA B. TEDROW, MD, MS

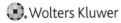 Wolters Kluwer

Philadelphia · Baltimore · New York · London
Buenos Aires · Hong Kong · Sydney · Tokyo

Executive Editor: Rebecca Gaertner
Senior Product Development Editor: Kristina Oberle
Production Project Manager: Bridgett Dougherty
Marketing Manager: Stephanie Kindlick
Senior Manufacturing Coordinator: Beth Welsh
Design Coordinator: Teresa Mallon
Production Service: Aptara, Inc.

© 2016 by Wolters Kluwer Health

9 8 7 6 5 4 3

Printed in China

Library of Congress Cataloging-in-Publication Data
Pocket cardiology : a companion to Pocket medicine / editor, Marc S. Sabatine ; authors, Marc P. Bonaca, Gregory D. Lewis, Michelle L. O'Donoghue, Usha B. Tedrow.
    p. ; cm. – (Pocket notebook)
Includes index.
ISBN 978-1-4511-9188-2 (alk. paper)
I. Sabatine, Marc S., editor. II. Pocket medicine. 5th edition. Complemented by (work):
III. Series: Pocket notebook.
[DNLM: 1. Cardiovascular Diseases–Handbooks. WG 39]
RC55
616–dc23

                                                            2015032058

CONTENTS

CONTRIBUTING AUTHORS

Marc P. Bonaca, MD, MPH
Investigator, TIMI Study Group
Associate Physician, Division of Cardiovascular Medicine, Brigham and Women's Hospital
Instructor in Medicine, Harvard Medical School

Gregory D. Lewis, MD
Director, Cardiology Intensive Care Unit; Director, Cardiopulmonary Exercise
    Laboratory; Medical Director, Mechanical Circulatory Support Program
Associate Physician, Cardiovascular Division, Massachusetts General Hospital
Assistant Professor of Medicine, Harvard Medical School

Michelle L. O'Donoghue, MD, MPH
Investigator, TIMI Study Group
Associate Physician, Division of Cardiovascular Medicine, Brigham and Women's Hospital
Affiliate Physician, Cardiology Division, Massachusetts General Hospital
Assistant Professor of Medicine, Harvard Medical School

Marc S. Sabatine, MD, MPH
Chairman, TIMI Study Group
Lewis Dexter, MD Distinguished Chair in Cardiovascular Medicine, Brigham and
    Women's Hospital
Affiliate Physician, Cardiology Division, Massachusetts General Hospital
Professor of Medicine, Harvard Medical School

Usha B. Tedrow, MD, MS
Director, Clinical Cardiac Electrophysiology Program
Director, Women and Arrhythmias Program
Physician, Division of Cardiovascular Medicine, Brigham and Women's Hospital
Associate Professor of Medicine, Harvard Medical School

PREFACE

With *Pocket Cardiology*, we now offer those taking care of patients with complex cardiovascular disease a focused and concise reference to aid them in their daily clinical care. *Pocket Cardiology* has been designed to either supplant the Cardiology section in *Pocket Medicine* or serve as a stand-alone handbook. *Pocket Cardiology* provides greatly expanded coverage of the latest treatment options for the major common cardiovascular diseases as well as new sections on advanced heart failure, vascular, and electrophysiology topics.

We have incorporated key references to the most recent high-tier reviews and important studies published right up to the time *Pocket Cardiology* went to press. We welcome any suggestions for further improvement. Although the recommendations herein are as evidence based as possible, sound clinical judgement must be applied to every scenario.

This book would not have been possible without the help of Melinda Cuerda, who shepherded the project from start to finish, with an incredible eye to detail to ensure that each page of this book was the very best it could be.

It is a privilege to take care of patients, especially when working with the house officers, fellows, and attendings at Brigham and Women's Hospital and the Massachusetts General Hospital. The rapid advances in cardiovascular medicine are truly amazing. We hope the information contained within *Pocket Cardiology* proves useful in your quest to deliver the best possible care to your patients.

MARC S. SABATINE, MD, MPH

ELECTROCARDIOGRAPHY

Approach *(a systematic approach is vital)*
- **Rate** (? tachy or brady)
- **Rhythm** (? P waves, ? relationship between P and QRS, ? regular)
- **Intervals** (PR, QRS, QT) and **axis** (? LAD or RAD)
- **Chamber abnormality** (? LAA and/or RAA, ? LVH and/or RVH)
- **QRST changes** (? Q waves, poor R-wave progression V_1–V_6, ST ↑/↓ or T-wave Δs)

Figure 1-1 QRS axis

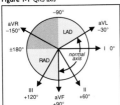

Left axis deviation (LAD)
- **Definition:** axis beyond −30° (S > R in lead II)
- **Etiologies:** LVH, LBBB, inferior MI, WPW
- **Left anterior fascicular block (LAFB):** LAD (−45 to −90°) *and* qR in aVL *and* QRS <120 msec *and* no other cause of LAD (eg, IMI)

Right axis deviation (RAD)
- **Definition:** axis beyond +90° (S > R in lead I)
- **Etiologies:** RVH, PE, COPD (usually not > +110°), septal defects, lateral MI, WPW
- **Left posterior fascicular block (LPFB):** RAD (90–180°) *and* rS in I & aVL *and* qR in III & aVF *and* QRS <120 msec *and* no other cause of RAD

Bundle Branch Blocks *(Circ 2009;119:e235)*		
Normal	V_1 V_6	Initial depol. is left-to-right across septum (r in V_1 & q in V_6; nb, absent in LBBB) followed by LV & RV free wall, with LV dominating (nb, RV depol. later and visible in RBBB).
RBBB		1. QRS ≥120 msec (110–119 = incomplete) 2. rSR' in R precordial leads (V_1,V_2) 3. Wide S wave in I and V_6 4. ± ST↓ or TWI in R precordial leads
LBBB		1. QRS ≥120 msec (110–119 = incomplete) 2. Broad, slurred, monophasic R in I, aVL, V_5–V_6 (± RS in V_5–V_6 if cardiomegaly) 3. Absence of Q in I, V_5 and V_6 (may have narrow q in aVL) 4. Displacement of ST & Tw opposite major QRS deflection 5. ± PRWP, LAD, Qw's in inferior leads

Bifascicular block: RBBB + LAFB/LPFB. Trifascicular block: bifascicular block + 1° AVB (nb, misnomer as 1° AVB involves AV node but no fascicle per se).

Prolonged QT interval *(NEJM 2008;358:169; www.torsades.org)*
- QT measured from beginning of QRS complex to end of T wave (measure longest QT)
- QT varies w/ HR → corrected w/ Bazett formula: QTc = QT/$\sqrt{RR}$ (RR in sec, can be estimated by 60/HR), overcorrects at high HR and undercorrects at low HR (nl QTc <440 msec ♂ and <460 msec ♀)
- Fridericia's formula preferred at very high or low HR: QTc = QT/$\sqrt[3]{RR}$
- QT prolongation a/w ↑ risk TdP (espec >500 msec); perform baseline/serial ECGs if using QT prolonging meds, no estab guidelines for stopping Rx if QT prolongs
- Etiologies:

  Antiarrhythmics: class Ia (procainamide, disopyramide), class III (amio, sotalol, dofet)
  Psych drugs: antipsychotics (phenothiazines, haloperidol, atypicals), Li, ? SSRI, TCA
  Antimicrobials: macrolides, quinolones, azoles, pentamidine, atovaquone, atazanavir
  Other: antiemetics (droperidol, 5-HT₃ antagonists), alfuzosin, methadone, ranolazine
  Electrolyte disturbances: hypoCa (nb, hyperCa a/w ↓ QT), ± hypoK, ? hypoMg
  Autonomic dysfxn: ICH (deep TWI), stroke, carotid endarterectomy, neck dissection
  Congenital (long QT syndrome): K, Na, & Ca channelopathies *(Circ 2013;127:126)*
  Misc: CAD, CMP, bradycardia, high-grade AVB, hypothyroidism, hypothermia, BBB

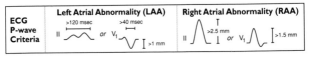

ECG P-wave Criteria	Left Atrial Abnormality (LAA)		Right Atrial Abnormality (RAA)	
	>120 msec	>40 msec	>2.5 mm	
	II	or V_1 >1 mm	II or V_1	>1.5 mm

Left ventricular hypertrophy (LVH) (Circ 2009;119:e251)
- Etiologies: HTN, AS/AI, HCMP, coarctation of aorta
- Criteria (affected by age, sex, race, BMI): Se <50%, Sp >85%; accuracy affected by age, sex, race, BMI)
  Romhilt-Estes point-score system (4 points = probable; 5 points = diagnostic):

Criteria	Points
Voltage (any of the following): R or S in limb leads ≥20 mm; S in V_1 or V_2 ≥30 mm; R in V_5 or V_6 ≥30 mm	3
ST-T displacement opposite to QRS deflection (either): • Pt not on digoxin • Pt on digoxin	3 1
Left atrial enlargement	3
Left axis deviation	2
QRS duration ≥90 msec	1
Delayed intrinsicoid deflection (QRS onset to R peak) in V_5 or V_6 >50 msec	1

Sokolow-Lyon: S in V_1 + R in V_5 or V_6 ≥35 mm or R in aVL ≥11 mm
Cornell: R in aVL + S in V_3 >28 mm in men or >20 mm in women
If LAD/LAFB, S in III + max (R+S) in precordium ≥30 mm

Right ventricular hypertrophy (RVH) (Circ 2009;119:e251)
- Etiologies: cor pulmonale, congenital (tetralogy, TGA, PS, ASD, VSD), MS, TR
- Criteria (all tend to be insensitive, but highly specific, except in COPD)
  R > S in V_1 or R in V_1 ≥7 mm, S in V_5 or V_6 ≥7 mm, drop in R/S ratio across precordium
  RAD ≥+110° (LVH + RAD or prominent S in V_5, V_6 → biventricular hypertrophy)

Ddx of dominant R wave in V_1 or V_2
- Ventricular enlargement: RVH (RAD, RAA, deep S waves in I, V_5, V_6); HCMP
- Myocardial injury: posterior MI (anterior Rw = posterior Qw; often with IMI)
- Abnormal depolarization: RBBB (QRS >120 msec, rSR'); WPW (↓ PR, δ wave, ↑ QRS)
- Other: dextroversion; Duchenne muscular dystrophy; lead misplacement; nl variant

Poor R wave progression (PRWP) (Am Heart J 2004;148:80)
- Definition: loss of anterior forces w/o frank Q waves (V_1–V_3); R wave in V_3 ≤3 mm
- Possible etiologies (nonspecific):
  old anteroseptal MI (usually w/ R wave V_3 ≤1.5 mm, ± persistent ST ↑ or TWI V_2 & V_3)
  cardiomyopathy
  LVH (delayed RWP with prominent left precordial voltage), RVH, COPD (which may also
   have RAA, RAD, limb lead QRS amplitude ≤5, $S_1S_{II}S_{III}$ w/ R/S ratio <1 in those leads)
  LBBB; WPW; clockwise rotation of the heart; lead misplacement; PTX

Pathologic Q waves
- Definition: ≥30 msec (≥20 msec V_2–V_3) or >25% height of R wave in that QRS complex
- Small (septal) q waves in I, aVL, V_5 & V_6 are nl, as can be isolated Qw in III, aVR, V_1
- "Pseudoinfarct" pattern may be seen in LBBB, infiltrative dis., HCMP, COPD, PTX, WPW
- In WPW, Qw pattern may help localize site of accessory pathway (Bundle of Kent)

ST elevation (STE) (NEJM 2003;349:2128; Circ 2009;119:e241 & e262)
- **Acute MI** (upward convexity ± TWI) or prior MI with persistent STE
- **Coronary spasm** (Prinzmetal's angina; transient STE in a coronary distribution)
- **Pericarditis** (diffuse, upward concavity STE; aVR PR ↓; Tw usually upright)
- **HCM, Takotsubo CMP, ventricular aneurysm, cardiac contusion**
- **Pulmonary embolism** (occ. STE V_1–V_3; classically w/ TWI V_1–V_4, RAD, RBBB, $S_1Q_3T_3$)
- **Repolarization abnormalities**
  LBBB (↑ QRS duration, STE discordant from QRS complex)
   dx of MI in setting of LBBB: Sgarbossa criteria (NEJM 1996;334:481)
    ≥1 mm STE concordant w/ QRS (Se 73%, Sp 92%)
    STD ≥1 mm V_1–V_3 (Se 25%, Sp 96%)
    STE ≥5 mm discordant w/ QRS (Se 31%, Sp 92%)
  LVH (↑ QRS amplitude)
  Brugada syndrome (rSR', downsloping STE V_1–V_2; Na channelopathy a/w SCD)
  Hyperkalemia (see below)
  Hypothermia: Osborn waves
   ⊕ deflection at J point, typically in R-precordial leads
   proportional to degree of hypothermia
- **aVR**: STE >1 mm a/w ↑ mortality in STEMI; STE aVR > V_1 a/w left main disease
- **Early repolarization**: most often seen in V_2–V_5 in young adults (JACC 2015;66:470)
  1–4 mm elev of peak of notch or start of slurred downstroke of R wave (ie, J point);
   ± up concavity of ST & large Tw (∴ ratio of STE/T wave <25%; may disappear w/ exercise)
  ? early repol in inf leads may be a/w ↑ risk of VF (NEJM 2009;361:2529; Circ 2011;124:2208)

ST depression (STD)
- **Myocardial ischemia** (± Tw abnl) or acute true posterior MI (V$_1$–V$_3$)
- Digitalis effect (downsloping ST ± Tw abnl, does *not* correlate w/ dig levels)
- Hypokalemia (± U wave)
- Repolarization abnl in a/w LBBB or LVH (usually in leads V$_5$, V$_6$, I, aVL)

T wave inversion (TWI; generally ≥1 mm; deep if ≥5 mm) (*Circ* 2009;119:e241)
- Ischemia or infarct; *Wellens' sign* (deep, symmetric precordial TWI) → proximal LCA lesion

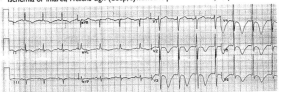

(Wellens' sign, from Cuculich PS and Kates AM. *The Washington Manual Cardiology Subspecialty Consult*, 3rd ed. Philadelphia: Wolters Kluwer Health, 2014:286.)

- Myopericarditis; CMP (Takotsubo, ARVC, apical HCM); MVP; PE (espec if TWI V$_1$–V$_4$)
- Repolarization abnl in a/w LVH/RVH ("strain pattern"), BBB
- Posttachycardia or postpacing
- Electrolyte, digoxin, PaO$_2$, PaCO$_2$, pH or core temperature disturbances
- Intracranial bleed ("cerebral T waves," usually w/ ↑ QT)
- Normal variant in children (V$_1$–V$_4$) and leads in which QRS complex predominantly ⊖

True posterior MI (posterior STE appearing as anterior STD)
- STD ± ↑ R wave in leads V$_1$–V$_4$ may correspond to acute posterior "ST-elevation" MI
- √ Posterior ECG leads; manage as a STEMI with rapid reperfusion

Anterior leads w/ ST depression   Placement of posterior ECG leads   Posterior leads s/ STE

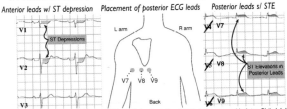

(Modified from Martindale JL, Brown DFM. *Rapid Interpretation of ECGs in Emergency Medicine*. Philadelphia: Lippincott Williams & Wilkins, 2012:364,376)

Low voltage
- QRS amplitude (R + S) <5 mm in all limb leads & <10 mm in all precordial leads
- Etiologies: COPD (precordial leads only), pericardial effusion, myxedema, obesity, pleural effusion, restrictive or infiltrative CMP, diffuse CAD

Electrolyte Abnormalities		
↑ K	Tented Tw, ↓ QT Small Pw, ↑ PR, AVB Wide QRS → sinusoidal pattern STE (typically V$_1$–V$_2$)	
↓ K	Flattened Tw U waves (⊕ deflection after T) ST depression Ectopy; ↑ QT & TdP	
↑ Ca	↓ QT, flattened Tw & Pw J point elevation	
↓ Ca	↑ QT; Tw Δs	

(ECGs modified from Wagner GS, Strauss DG. *Marriott's Practical Electrocardiography*, 12th ed. Philadelphia: Lippincott Williams & Wilkins, 2014)

CHEST PAIN

Disorder	Typical Characteristics & Diagnostic Studies
Cardiac Causes	
ACS (15–25% of chest pain in ED)	Substernal pressure radiating to neck, jaw, arm. ± Dyspnea, diaphoresis, N/V; a/w exertion; ↓ w/ NTG or rest; however, not reliable indicator (*Annals EM* 2005;45:581). ± ECG Δs: STE, STD, TWI, Qw. ± ↑ Troponin.
Pericarditis & myopericarditis	Sharp pain → trapezius, ↑ w/ respiration, ↓ w/ sitting forward. ± Pericardial friction rub. ECG Δs (diffuse STE & PR ↓, opposite in aVR) ± pericardial effusion. If myocarditis, same as above + ↑ Tn and ± s/s HF and ↓ EF.
Aortic dissection	Abrupt-onset severe tearing, knifelike pain (absence ⊖ LR 0.3), ant or post midscapular. HTN or HoTN. ± Asymmetric (>20 mmHg) BP or pulse deficit (⊕ LR 5.7), focal neuro deficit (⊕ LR >6), AI, widened mediastinum on CXR (absence ⊖ LR 0.3); false lumen on imaging. (*JAMA* 2002;287:2262)
Pulmonary Causes	
Pneumonia	Pleuritic; dyspnea, fever, cough, sputum. ↑ RR, crackles. CXR infiltrate.
Pleuritis	Sharp, pleuritic pain. ± Pleuritic friction rub.
PTX	Sudden onset, sharp pleuritic pain. Hyperresonance, ↓ BS. PTX on CXR.
PE	Sudden onset pleuritic pain. ↑ RR & HR, ↓ S_aO_2, ECG Δs (sinus tach, RAD, RBBB, $S_IQ_{III}T_{III}$, TWI V_1–V_4, occ STE V_1–V_3). ⊕ CTA or V/Q.
Pulm HTN	Exertional pressure, DOE. ↓ S_aO_2, loud P_2, RV heave, right S_3 and/or S_4.
GI Causes	
Esophageal reflux	Substernal burning, acid taste in mouth, water brash. ↑ by meals, recumbency; ↓ by antacids. EGD, manometry, pH monitoring.
Esoph spasm	Intense substernal pain. ↑ by swallowing, ↓ by NTG/CCB. Manometry.
Mallory-Weiss	Esophageal tear precipitated by vomiting. EGD.
Boerhaave syndrome	Esoph. rupture typically precipitated by vomiting. Severe pain, ↑ w/ swallowing. Palpable SC emphysema; mediastinal air on chest CT.
PUD	Epigastric pain, relieved by antacids. ± GIB. EGD, ± *H. pylori* test.
Biliary dis.	RUQ pain, N/V. ↑ by fatty foods. RUQ U/S; ↑ LFTs.
Pancreatitis	Epigastric/back discomfort. ↑ amylase & lipase; abd CT.
Musculoskeletal and Miscellaneous Causes	
Costochond	Localized sharp pain. ↑ w/ movement. Reproduced by palpation.
Zoster	Intense unilateral pain. Pain may precede dermatomal rash.
Anxiety	"Tightness," dyspnea, palpitations, other somatic symptoms

(*Braunwald's Heart Disease*, 10th ed, 2014)

Initial approach
- **Focused history:** quality & severity of pain; location & radiation; provoking & palliating factors; intensity at onset; duration, frequency & pattern; setting in which it occurred; associated sx; cardiac hx and risk factors

Pain Feature	Classic for ACS	Atypical for ACS
Quality	Pressure (⊕ LR 1.3), tightness, "Levine" sign (clenched fist over chest), squeezing, fullness, heavy weight, more than prior angina or ≈ prior MI (⊕ LR 1.8)	Sharp (⊕ LR 0.3)
Region/ radiation	Substernal, radiating to L or R arm or shoulder (⊕ LR 2.3–4.7), jaw, teeth, neck	Small area, points w/ 1 finger, radiation to back
Provocation	Exertion (⊕ LR 2.4; but may be absent)	Pleuritic, positional or w/ palp (⊕ LR ≤0.3), eating
Associated sx	Diaphoresis (⊕ LR 2.0), N/V (⊕ LR 1.9), dyspnea	

(*JAMA* 2005;294:2623)

- **Targeted exam:** VS (including BP in both arms), cardiac gallops, murmurs or rubs; signs of vascular disease (carotid or femoral bruits, ↓ pulses), signs of heart failure; lung & abdominal exam; chest wall exam for reproducibility of pain
- **12-lead ECG:** obtain w/in 10 min; c/w priors & obtain serial ECGs. In addition, consider: *posterior leads* (V_7–V_9; remove V_4–V_6 and place in post axillary, mid-clavic & L paraspinal position) useful to ✓ for posterior STEMI if hx c/w ACS but stnd ECG unrevealing, esp if ST ↓V_1–V_4 (ant ischemia vs post STEMI) or R/S V_1–V_2 >1 *R-sided leads* (place V_3–V_6 in mirror image position on R side of chest) in inferior STEMI to detect RV involvement

- **CXR**; other imaging (echo, PE CTA, etc.) as indicated based on H&P and initial testing
- **Biomarkers** (see below): Tn preferred biomarker, ✓ at baseline & 3–6 h after sx onset

Biomarkers

- **Troponin:** level >99th %ile w/ rise & fall in approp. setting is dx of MI; >95% Se, 90% Sp
  Detectable 1–6 h after injury, peaks 24 h, may remain elevated for 7–14 d in STEMI
  Tn may be ↑ in CKD in absence of ACS, ∴ add CK-MB/serial Tn for confirmation
  Sensitive Tn assays: 98% Se, 90% Sp, 75% PPV, 99% NPV w/in 3 h of admit to ED, 82%
  Se & 95% NPV at time of admission to ED (JAMA 2011;306:2684)
  High-sensitivity Tn assays quantify Tn in majority of healthy individ.; prog value in asx
  general pop., stable CAD & DM (NEJM 2009;361:2538 & 2015;373:610; JAMA 2010;304:2503)
- **CK-MB:** less Se & Sp than Tn for dx of MI
  Sources include skeletal muscle, tongue, diaphragm, intestine, uterus, prostate
  CK-MB relative index (ratio of CK-MB to CK) >2.5–3 suggests cardiac vs skel. muscle
  CK-MB begins to rise 4–6 h post MI (may take 12 h) and returns to baseline w/in 36–48 h
  May aid in gauging timing of MI (⊕ Tn & ⊖ CK-MB suggests MI several days ago)
  May help dx reinfarction if Tn already elevated; however, Tn should ↑ as well
- **Myoglobin & heart-type fatty acid binding protein** are smaller molecules that may
  appear in circulation as early as 30 min after MI, but lack of specificity limits utility
- **D-dimer:** low level useful to r/o PE (qv) and aortic dissection (qv)
- **B-type natriuretic peptide (BNP):** elevations not specific for ACS but suggest ↑ ventricular
  wall stress seen not only in decompensated HF, but also ACS & PE

Interpretation of elevated cardiac biomarkers (troponin or CK-MB)

- Does it reflect true myocardial injury? Almost always the case for Tn; CK-MB less specific.
- If myocardial injury, what is the pathobiology? Ddx includes:
  MI (injury due to ischemia): rise and/or fall in cardiac biomarker (preferably Tn)
  >99th %ile w/ ≥1 of the following:
  1) sx of ischemia
  2) new Qw
  3) new ST∆ or LBBB
  4) intracoronary thrombus
  5) imaging evidence of new loss of myocardium or regional wall motion abnl
  non-ischemic injury (eg, myocarditis/toxic CMP, cardiac contusion)
  multifactorial (eg, PE, sepsis, severe HF, renal failure, Takotsubo, infiltrative disease)
- If MI, what type? (Circ 2012;126:2020)

Type	Descriptor	Features
1	Spontaneous	Pathologic process in wall of coronary artery (eg, plaque rupture) resulting in intraluminal thrombus
2	Supply–demand mismatch not due to ∆ in CAD	Mismatch due to, eg, ↑↑ or ↓↓ HR or BP, profound anemia or hypoxemia, coronary vasospasm, HCM, severe AS
3	Sudden cardiac death	
4a	Related to PCI	Tn >5x 99th %ile or >20% rise if already elevated + ≥1 MI clinical/imaging criteria above
4b	Stent thrombosis	
5	Related to CABG	Tn >10x 99th %ile + new Qw or LBBB, angio confirmation, or new wall motion abnl

- Classification important as antithrombotic Rx relevant for type 1 but not type 2 MI,
  whereas anti-ischemic Rx (↑ O$_2$ supply & ↓ demand) particularly important for type 2

Early noninvasive imaging (also see noninvasive evaluation of CAD)

- If low prob of ACS (eg, ⊖ ECG & Tn) & stable → noninvasive fxnal or imaging test
- Treadmill electrocardiography: can be performed after 6–8 h of evaluation
- Radionuclide imaging in Pts who cannot exercise or have uninterpretable ECG
- Can perform acute rest perfusion imaging if ongoing or recent (w/in 2 h) pain
  (⊖ scan r/o ischemia; ⊕ scan could represent ischemia or infarct, need pain-free
  rest images)
- Echo (w/ or w/o stress) to assess for regional wall motion abnl; interpretation difficult
  in those w/ prior MI
- Coronary CT angio (CCTA): NPV 98% for signif CAD, but PPV 35% for ACS; helpful
  to r/o CAD if low-intermed prob of ACS. CCTA vs noninvasive fxnal test for ischemia → ↓ time to dx & LOS, but ↑ probability of cath/PCI, contrast exposure &
  ↑ radiation (NEJM 2012;366:1393 & 367:299; JACC 2013;61:880)
- "Triple r/o" CT angiogram for CAD, PE, AoD

NONINVASIVE EVALUATION OF CAD

Stress testing (*Circ* 2007;115:1464; *JACC* 2012;60:1828)
- **Indications:** dx CAD, evaluate Δ in clinical status in Pt w/ known CAD, risk stratify s/p ACS, evaluate exercise tolerance, localize ischemia (imaging required)
- **Contraindications** (*Circ* 2002;106:1883; & 2012;126:2465)
  Absolute: AMI w/in 48 h, high-risk UA, acute PE, severe sx AS, uncontrolled HF, uncontrolled arrhythmias, myopericarditis, acute aortic dissection
  Relative: left main CAD, mod valvular stenosis, severe HTN, HCMP, high-degree AVB, severe electrolyte abnl

Exercise tolerance test
- Generally preferred if patient can exercise to a meaningful level; Se ~65%, Sp ~80%
- Typically via treadmill

Protocol	Description
Standard Bruce	↑ speed & incline q3min until 85% max predicted HR or sxs
Modified Bruce	Adds two stages at start that require less work than standard Bruce stage 1; consider in sedentary/deconditioned Pt
Submaximal	Stop earlier (eg, 70% max predicted HR or 5 METs or any anginal sx); consider if recent MI

- Stationary cycle or arm ergometry (lower max workload) if Pt cannot walk
- Hold anti-ischemic meds (eg, nitrates, βB, CCB, ranolazine) if trying to dx obstructive CAD, but continue meds when assessing if Pt ischemic on current med regimen

Pharmacologic stress test (nb, requires imaging as ECG not interpretable)
- Use if unable to exercise, low exerercise tolerance, or recent MI. Se & Sp ≈ exercise.
- Preferred if LBBB or V-paced, as higher prob of false ⊕ exercise imaging (typically reversible or fixed anteroseptal defect).
- **Coronary vasodilator:** diffuse coronary arteriolar vasodilation → relative "coronary steal" from vessels w/ fixed epicardial disease. Reveals CAD, but *not if Pt ischemic w/ exercise.* Options include:
  Adenosine or dipyridamole (↓ adenosine reuptake). Side effects: flushing, bradycardia & AVB, dyspnea & bronchospasm.
  Selective A_{2A} receptor agonist (eg, regadenoson): less flushing, dyspnea, bronchospasm
  Longer half-life of dipyridamole & regadenoson allow to be combined w/ exercise
  Avoid caffeine (adenosine receptor antagonist) w/in 12 h of test. Conversely, can use aminophylline to reverse effects of these agents.
  Contraindic: HoTN, sick sinus, high-degree AVB, bronchospasm (selective agents safer)
- **Chronotropes/inotropes** (more physiologic): dobutamine (may precip tachyarrhythmia)

Imaging for stress test (see Photo Inserts)
- Use if uninterpretable ECG (V-paced, LBBB, resting ST ↓ >1 mm, digoxin, LVH, WPW), after indeterminate ECG test, or if pharmacologic test
- Use when need to localize ischemia (often used if prior coronary revasc)
- Ideally use exercise as stress modality rather than pharmacologic
- **Radionuclide myocardial perfusion imaging** w/ images obtained at rest & w/ stress
  SPECT (eg, ^{99m}Tc-sestamibi): Se ~85%, Sp ~80%
  PET (rubidium-82): Se ~90%, Sp ~85%
  ECG-gated imaging allows assessment of LV fxn (including regional systolic wall thickening or lack thereof as a sign of ischemia/infarction)
- **Echo** (exercise or dobuta): Se ~85%, Sp ~85%; no radiation; operator dependent
- Cardiac MRI (w/ pharmacologic stress) another option with excellent Se & Sp

Test results
- **HR** (must achieve ≥85% of max pred HR [220 − age] for exer. test to be dx), **BP** response, peak **double product** (HR × BP; nl >20k), HR recovery (HR$_{peak}$ − HR$_{1\,min\,later}$; nl >12)
- **Max exercise capacity** achieved (METS or min)
- Occurrence of **symptoms** (at what level of exertion and similarity to presenting sx)
- **ECG Δs:** downsloping or horizontal ST ↓ (≥1 mm) 80 ms after QRS predictive of CAD
  upsloping ST ↓ w/ rapid return to baseline usually due to ↑ HR & atrial repol artifact
  lead V$_5$ most sensitive; Δ isolated to inferior leads may be artifact
  location of ST ↓ does *not* localize ischemic territory
  STE: highly predictive of CAD & localizes; in aVR suggests LM CAD; nonspecific if in leads w/ prior Qw
- **Duke treadmill score** = exercise min − (5 × max ST dev) − (4 × angina index)
  [angina index = 0 none, 1 nonlimiting sxs, 2 limiting sxs]

Category	CAD	1-y mort	5-y survival
Low risk (≥5)	60% w/o signif stenosis	<1%	97%
Moderate risk (−10 to 4)	31% w/ 3VD or LM	2–3%	90%
High risk (≤−11)	74% w/ 3VD or LM	≥5%	65%

- **Imaging:** radionuclide defects or echocardiographic regional wall motion abnormalities
  reversible defect = ischemia; fixed defect = infarct; transient isch dilation = severe CAD
  false ⊕: breast → ant "defect" and diaphragm → inf "defect"
  false ⊖ may be seen if balanced (eg, 3VD) ischemia (global ↓ perfusion w/o regional Δs)

High-risk test results
- ECG: ST ↓ ≥2 mm or ≥1 mm in stage 1 or in ≥5 leads or ≥5 min in recovery; STE; VT
- Physiologic: ↓ or fail to ↑ BP, <4 METS, angina during exercise, Duke score ≤ −11; ↓ EF
- Radionuclide: ≥1 lg or ≥2 mod. reversible defects, transient LV cavity dilation, ↑ lung uptake
- High-risk test has PPV ~50% for LM or 3VD, ∴ consider coronary angio

Myocardial viability (Circ 2008;117:103; Eur Heart J 2011;31:2984 & 2011;32:810)
- Viable myocardium = dysfxn at rest, but not scarred and has potential for recovery
- Goal: identify hibernating or stunned myocardium that could regain fxn after revasc

Viability Test	Sens	Spec	Mechanism
MRI	~85%	~75%	Assesses cellular integrity
PET	~90%	~65%	Assesses cell metabolism
Dobut stress echo	~80%	~80%	Assesses contractile reserve
Myocard contrast echo	~85%	~50%	Assesses cellular integrity
Thallium: rest-redistrib or stress-reinjection	~85%	~55%	Assesses cellular integrity (K+ analogue taken up by Na/K-ATPase)
Technetium-MIBI	~85%	~65%	Assesses cellular integrity (requires intact mitochondria)

- However, in Pts w/ ↓ EF, presence of viability did not identify differential clinical benefit from CABG vs med Rx (NEJM 2011;364:1617)

Coronary CT angio (CCTA; NEJM 2008;359:2324; Circ 2010;121:2509)
- High NPV to r/o CAD, but low PPV
- In Pts presenting with CP, presence of plaque sensitive (100%) but not specific (54%)
  for ACS, ∴ NPV 100%, PPV 17% (JACC 2009;53:1642). CCTA vs noninvasive fxnal test
  for ischemia → ↓ time to dx & LOS, but ↑ probability of cath/PCI, contrast exposure
  & ↑ radiation (NEJM 2012;366:1393 & 367:299; JACC 2013;61:880).
- In sx outPt, CCTA vs fxnal testing led to more radiation, coronary angiography &
  revascularization, but no difference in clinical outcomes (PROMISE NEJM 2015;372:1291)
- CCTA images may be limited if: HR >60–70 bpm, irregular rhythm, calcium deposition
  or stents (may create artifact), inability to breath hold 5 sec, vessel diameter <1.5 mm.
  Image quality best at slower & regular HR (? give βB if possible, goal HR 55–60).
- Useful for assessing patency of bypass grafts

MRI angiography (Lancet 2012;379:453)
- Unlike CCTA, does not require iodinated contrast, HR control or radiation exposure.
  Can also assess LV fxn, enhancement (early = microvasc obstruction; late = MI).
  Limitations: cost, operator-dependent, long duration, ↓ spatial resolution.
- In head-to-head comparisons, CMRI and CCTA appear to have grossly comparable
  sensitivity and specificity (JACC 2005;46:92; Annals 2006;145:207)

Coronary artery calcium score (NEJM 2012;366:294; JAMA 2012;308:788)
- Quantifies extent of calcium; thus estimates plaque burden (but not % coronary stenosis)
- Compared w/ CCTA, CAC score assessment requires lower radiation exposure (1–2 mSv)
- CAC sensitive (91%) but not specific (49%) for presence of CAD; high NPV to r/o CAD

CAC Score	Suggested plaque burden
0	No disease
1–99	Mild disease
100–399	Moderate disease
>400	Severe disease

- ? value as screening test to r/o CAD in sx Pt (CACS <100 → 3% probability of signif
  CAD; but interpretation affected by age, gender)
- May provide incremental value to clinical scores for risk stratification (JAMA 2004;291:210).
  ACC/AHA guidelines note CAC assessment is reasonable in asx Pts w/ intermed risk
  (10–20% 10-y Framingham risk; ? value if 6–10% 10-y risk) (Circ 2010;122:e584).

STABLE ISCHEMIC HEART DISEASE

Epidemiology is U.S. (Circ 2015;131:e29)
- Prevalence: 20–39 y: <1%; 40–59 y: 5-6%; 60–79 y: 21% in ♂ & 11% in ♀; ≥80 y: 35% in ♂ & 19% in ♀; lifetime risk after age 40: 50% in men & 32% in women
- Ischemic heart disease (IHD) remains leading cause of death in both men & women

Workup (Circ 2012;126:e354)
- Initiate workup if suspected new dx of IHD or Δ in clinical status
- H&P, ECG (looking for ischemic or prior infarct Δs such as Qw, PRWP, ST or Tw abnl)

Pretest Likelihood of CAD (%) (NEJM 1979;300:1350; Annals 1993;118:81)					
	Nonanginal (≤1 sx)		**Atypical angina (2 sx)**		**Typical angina (all 3 sx)**	
Age	**Men**	**Women**	**Men**	**Women**	**Men**	**Women**
35	3 ↔ 35	1 ↔ 19	8 ↔ 59	2 ↔ 39	30 ↔ 88	10 ↔ 78
45	9 ↔ 47	2 ↔ 22	21 ↔ 70	5 ↔ 43	51 ↔ 92	20 ↔ 79
55	23 ↔ 59	4 ↔ 21	45 ↔ 79	10 ↔ 47	80 ↔ 95	38 ↔ 82
65	49 ↔ 69	9 ↔ 29	71 ↔ 86	20 ↔ 51	93 ↔ 97	56 ↔ 84

Classic angina sx: substernal chest pain, provoked by exertion, relieved by rest or NTG. W/in each cell, 1ˢᵗ # is % for Pt w/o risk factors; 2ⁿᵈ is for Pt w/ DM, smoking, & hyperchol.

- **Noninvasive testing** (qv) if intermediate risk (ie, >10–20% & <80–90%). If Pt has low prob, then ↑ risk false ⊕; if very high prob, ∴ test does not adeq r/o CAD, ∴ consider cor angio.
- **Coronary angio** if: high-risk noninv results (qv); very high pretest prob; refract angina; uncertain dx after noninvasive testing (& compelling need to determine dx), occupational need for definitive dx (eg, pilot) or inability to undergo noninvasive testing; survivor of SCD or life-threatening vent. arrhythmia; unexplained heart failure or ↓ EF; suspected spasm or nonatherosclerotic cause of ischemia (eg, anomalous coronary)

Optimal medical therapy (OMT) (Circ 2012;126:e354 & 2014;130:1749; HTN 2015;65:1372)
- **ASA** 75–162 mg/d; **βB** for 3 y post MI or if ↓ EF; **statin** (typically high intensity; see "Lipids")
- **ACEI** (or ARB) if HTN, DM, CKD or ↓ EF
- Risk factor targets: BP <140/90 (consider <130/80 if prior MI), HbA_{1c} 7–9% (<7% if long life expect.), BMI 18.5–24.9 kg/m²
- Smoking cessation; influenza vaccine
- Diet: ↑ veg, fruits, whole grains; ↓ sweets, sugar-sweetened bevs & red meat; sat fat 5–6% total cals, trans fat <1% total cals, chol <200 mg/d; Na ≤2400 mg/d (ideally ≤1500 mg/d)
- Exercise: ~40 min moderate-to-vigorous physical activity 3–4x/wk

Medical therapies for symptomatic relief (Circ 2012;126:e354)
- **Beta blockers** 1ˢᵗ-line therapy
- **CCB** (verap/dilt or long-acting dihydro) or **long-acting nitrates**: add-on or if βB intolerant
- **Ranolazine** (↓ late inward Na+ current to ↓ myocardial demand): add-on or if βB intolerant

Coronary revascularization (Circ 2011;124:e574)
- If unacceptable angina despite max tolerated med Rx or if potential to improve survival
- OMT should be initial focus if stable & w/o critical anatomy & w/ normal EF
- Older studies showed survival benefit w/ revasc (CABG) vs med Rx (pre-statin era) if: LM (≥50% stenosis), 3VD (≥70% stenoses) espec if ↓ EF, 2VD w/ critical prox LAD, ? 1–2 VD w/ large area of viable, ischemic myocardium

Recent Studies of Revascularization in Modern Era of OMT			
Compare	**Trial**	**Pts**	**Result**
PCI vs OMT	COURAGE[a]	1–3VD, EF >30%	PCI does not ↓ D/MI; faster sx resolution
	FAME-II[b]	≥1VD w/ FFR (qv) ≤0.8	PCI ↑ peri-PCI MI, but then 44% ↓ death/ spont MI; ? greater benefit if FFR <0.65
CABG vs OMT	STITCH[c]	EF ≤35% (majority w/ 3VD)	CABG 20% ↓ CV death, no Δ in all-cause mortality
CABG vs PCI	SYNTAX[d]	3VD or LM	CABG ↓ D/MI & revasc but ± ↑ stroke High SYNTAX/SYNTAX II score[g] ID's those who benefit most from CABG
	PRECOMBAT[e]	LM	PCI ? noninferior but ↑ repeat revasc
	FREEDOM[f]	DM w/ ≥2VD	CABG ↓ D/MI, but ↑ stroke

[a]NEJM 2007;356:1503; [b]NEJM 2014;371:1208; [c]NEJM 2011;364:1607; [d]Lancet 2013;381:629 & 639; [e]NEJM 2011;364:1718; [f]NEJM 2012;367:2375; [g]www.syntaxscore.com

- LM or 3VD: CABG, espec if ↓ EF or DM; consider PCI if SYNTAX score ≤22 & high surg risk
- 2VD w/ prox LAD, ↓ EF, or extensive ischemia: CABG (espec if DM) or ? PCI
- ? 1VD (low FFR) w/ prox LAD + either ↓ EF or extensive ischemia: PCI or CABG (w/ LIMA)
- Exp't device to narrow coronary sinus ↓ angina (NEJM 2015;372:517)

LIPID DISORDERS

Measurements

- Lipoproteins = lipids (cholesteryl esters & triglycerides) + phospholipids + proteins
  include: chylomicrons, VLDL, IDL, LDL, HDL, Lp(a)
- Measure after 12-h fast; LDL is typically calculated w/ Friedewald equation:
  LDL-C = TC − HDL-C − (TG/5) [last term assumes TG:VLDL ratio = 5:1]; underestim.
  if TG >400 or LDL-C <70 mg/dL (*JAMA* 2013;310:2061); ∴ directly measure LDL-C
  Non–HDL-C (TC − HDL-C) and apoB are alternative nonfasting measures of risk
  Lipid levels stable up to 24 h after ACS and other acute illnesses, then ↓ and may
  take 6 wk to return to nl
- Metabolic syndrome (≥3 of following): waist ≥40" (♂) or ≥35" (♀); TG ≥150; HDL <40 mg/dL
  (♂) or <50 mg/dL (♀); BP ≤130/85 mmHg; fasting glc ≤100 mg/dL (*Circ* 2009;120:1640)
- Lp(a) = LDL particle bound to apo(a) via apoB; genetic variants a/w MI (*NEJM* 2009;361:2518)

Primary dyslipidemias

- Familial hypercholesterolemia (FH, 1:500): defective LDL receptor; ↑↑ chol, nl TG; ↑ CAD
- Familial defective apoB100 (1:1000): similar to FH
- Familial combined hyperlipidemia (1:200): polygenic; ↑ chol, ↑ TG, ↓ HDL; ↑ CAD
- Familial dysbetalipoproteinemia (1:10,000): ↑ chol & TG; xanthomas; ↑ CAD
- Familial hypertriglyceridemia (FHTG, 1:500): ↑ TG, ± ↑ chol, ↓ HDL, pancreatitis

Secondary Dyslipidemias	
Category	**Disorders**
Endocrinopathies	Type 2 diabetes (↑ TG, ↓ HDL); lipodystrophy (↑ TG) Hypothyroidism (↑ LDL, ↑ TG); hyperthyroidism (↓ LDL) Cushing's syndrome & exogenous steroids (↑ LDL, ↑ TG)
Renal diseases	Renal failure (↑ LDL, ↑ TG); nephrotic syndrome (↑ LDL, ↑ TG)
Hepatic diseases	Cholestasis, PBC (↑ LDL); liver failure (↓ LDL); acute hepatitis (↑ TG)
Lifestyle	Obesity, sat & trans fat (↑ TG, ↓ HDL, ↑ LDL); sedentary lifestyle (↓ HDL); alcohol (↑ TG, ↑ HDL); tobacco (↓ HDL); anorexia (↑ LDL); very low-fat diet, high-refined-carb diet (↑ TG); preg (↑ LDL; ↑ TG)
Medications	Thiazides (↑ LDL, ↑ TG); βB (except carvedilol, ↑ TG, ↓ HDL); prote- ase inhib (↑ TG); estrogens (↑ TG, ↑ HDL); androgens (↓ HDL); cyclo- sporine, amiodarone (↑ LDL); bile acid sequestrants, protease inhib, retin. acid, sirolimus, raloxifene, tamoxifen (↑ TG)

Physical exam findings

- Tendon xanthomas: seen on Achilles, elbows and hands; implies LDL >300 mg/dL
- Eruptive xanthomas: pimple-like lesions on extensor surfaces; implies TG >1000 mg/dL
- Xanthelasma: yellowish streaks on eyelids seen in various dyslipidemias
- Corneal arcus: common in older adults, imply hyperlipidemia in young Pts

Drug Treatment				
Drug	**↓ LDL**	**↑ HDL**	**↓ TG**	**Side effects/comments**
Statins	20–60%	5–10%	10–25%	Doubling of dose → 6% further ↓ LDL. ↑ ALT in 0.5–3% (dose-dependent); ✓ before starting and then after as clinically indicated Myalgias <10% (not always ↑ CK), myositis 0.5%, rhabdo <0.1%. risk dose-dependent ↑ risk of DM (may be related to LDL-R; *JAMA* 2015;313:1029); screen if risk factors
Ezetimibe	15–20%	—	—	Well tolerated; typically w/ statin
Fibrates	5–15%	5–15%	35–50%	Myopathy risk ↑ w/ statin (gemfibrozil > fenofi- brate). Dyspepsia, gallstones, ↑ Cr. ✓ renal fxn at baseline, 3 mo, q6mo.
Niacin	10–25%	~30%	40%	Flushing (less w/ sustained release; ASA preRx may ↓), hyperglycemia, ↑ UA. ✓ renal fxn, UA, glc ± HbA1c at baseline and q6mo or w/ uptitration.
Resins	20%	3–5%	↑	Bloating, binds other meds
Ω-3 FA	5% ↑	3%	25–50%	Dyspepsia, diarrhea, skin Δs, bleeding
PCSK9 inhibitors	40–65%	5–10%	15–25%	mAb inj SC q2w or q4w (*Lancet* 2012;380:2007 & *JACC* 2015;65:2638)
CETP inhibitors	~30%	140%	5–10%	*Investigational* (*NEJM* 2010;363:2406; *Lancet* 2015;386:452)

Treatment of LDL-C (Lancet 2014;384:607)
- **Statins:** every 1 mmol (39 mg/dL) ↓ LDL-C → 22% ↓ major vascular events (CV death, MI, stroke, revasc) in individuals w/ & w/o CAD (Lancet 2010;376:1670); ∴ mainstay of therapy as potent, safe and well-tolerated
- Consistent CV benefit even in individuals starting w/ LDL-C ≤60 mg/dL (JACC 2011;57:1666)
- No clear evidence to date to suggest any harm from achieving very low LDL-C levels
- Elevated hs-CRP may identify Pts who derive ↑ benefit (NEJM 2001;344:1959 & 2008;359:2195)
- Similar clinical benefit also seen w/ some older nonstatin Rxs (resins, fibrates, niacin) when sufficiently lowered LDL-C (JACC 2005;46:1855)
- **Ezetimibe:** ↓ major vascular events incl MI & stroke when added to statin post-ACS, w/ magnitude of benefit consistent w/ LDL-statin relationship (IMPROVE-IT, NEJM 2015;372:2387)
- **PCSK9 inhibitors:** ~60% ↓ LDL on top of statin, as monoRx, and in FH (EHJ 2014;35:2249); prelim data w/ encouraging ↓ CV outcomes (NEJM 2015;372:1500), definitive trials ongoing

Treatment of HDL-C (Lancet 2014;384:618)
- Low levels of HDL-C associated w/ ↑ risk of MI
- However, Mendelian randomization studies do not support causal role (Lancet 2011;380:572)
- **Niacin:** in Pts w/ well-controlled LDL-C (<80 mg/dL) on a statin, minimally ↓ LDL, modestly ↑ HDL, and did not ↓ CV events (NEJM 2011;365:2255 & 2014;371:203)
- **CETP inhibitors:** one that ↑ HDL-C by 25% did not lead to clinical benefit in Pts w/ well-controlled LDL-C on a statin (NEJM 2012;367:2089); CV outcomes trials of inhibitors that ↑ HDL-C by 140% and ↓ LDL-C by ~30% ongoing (NEJM 2010;363:2406; JAMA 2011;306:2099)

Treatment of hypertriglyceridemia (Lancet 2014;384:626)
- Reasonable to treat very high levels (>500–1000 mg/dL) to ↓ risk of pancreatitis
- High levels of TG associated w/ ↑ risk of MI, but whether causal remains debated
- **Fibrates** (gemfibrozil & fenofibrate): mixed data in terms of ↓ vascular events, ? greater benefit if high TG (Circ 1992;85:37; NEJM 1999;341:410; Lancet 2005;366:1849; NEJM 2010;362:1563)
- **Fish oil** (containing Ω-3 fatty acids EPA & DHA): recent meta-analyses suggest supplementation w/o meaningful effect on CV events (JAMA 2012;308:1024)
- APOC3 inhibitors under study and ↓ TG by up to ~70% (NEJM 2015;373:438)

Treatment of Lp(a)
- Consider ↓ to <50 mg/dL w/ niacin in intermed- to high-risk Pts (EHJ 2010;31:2844–53); however, benefit unclear espec if LDL-C well controlled (JACC 2014;63:520)

Guidelines (Circ 2014;129(Suppl 2):S1)
- Focus now on statin strategies, rather than achieving LDL-C goals
- Clinical atherosclerotic CV disease (ASCVD) includes h/o ACS, stable angina, arterial revasc, stroke, TIA, or PAD presumed to be of atherosclerotic origin
- 10-y CV Risk Score for CHD or stroke based on age, sex, race, SBP, TC, LDL, DM, tobacco, BP Rx; http://my.americanheart.org/cvriskcalculator
- Additional risk factors to consider include: LDL-C ≥160 mg/dL, genetic hyperlipid., FHx premature ASCVD, hsCRP >2 mg/L, CAC score ≥300 or ≥75th %ile, ABI <0.9.

2013 ACC/AHA Guideline of Treatment of Blood Cholesterol		
Population	**10-y CV risk**	**Statin Recommendation**
Clinical ASCVD (ie, 2° prevention)	n/a	High intensity. If age >75 y, eval risk-benefit for high vs moderate intensity
LDL-C ≥190 mg/dL	n/a	High intensity
DM (type 1 or 2); age 40–75 y	≥7.5%	High intensity
	<7.5%	Moderate intensity
Age 40–75 y (and none of the above)	≥7.5%	High or moderate intensity
	5–<7.5%	Reasonable to offer moderate intensity
	<5%	Consider statin if additional risk factor

- If statin intolerant or LDL-C remains elevated despite high-intensity statin (as well as reinforcement of med adherence, lifestyle changes and exclusion of 2° causes of dyslipidemia) nonstatin LDL-lowering therapies remain reasonable
- If Pt does not tolerate high-intensity statin, consider dose reduction before d/c statin

Statin Doses & LDL-C Reduction								
Intensity	**↓ LDL-C**	**Rosuva**	**Atorva**	**Simva**	**Prava**	**Lova**	**Fluva**	**Pitava**
High	≥50%	20–40	40–80	(80)				
Mod	30–50%	5–10	10–20	20–40	40–80	40	80	2–4
Low	<30%			10	10–20	20	20–40	1

Doses are in mg. Simva 80 mg has ↑ myopathy risk and should not be used unless dose already tolerated >12 mo.

ANGIOGRAPHY, PCI, & CABG

Precath checklist
- Document peripheral arterial exam (radial, femoral, DP, PT pulses; bruits); if plan for radial artery access, ✓ palmar arch intact (eg, w/ pulse oximetry & plethysmography), although value remains unproven (JACC 2014;63:1833)
- Ensure Pt can lie flat for several hours
- ✓ CBC, PT-INR (ideally ≤1.5), & Cr; blood bank sample
- NPO >6 h; IVF if appropriate (± bicarb; acetylcysteine no longer rec; see "CIAKI")

Vascular access
- Femoral artery commonly used; high puncture ↑ risk of retroperitoneal bleed; low puncture ↑ risk of peripheral arterial complic.; can access a synthetic graft if a few months old
- Radial artery: 33% ↓ major bleeding, trend to 15% ↓ in MACE & 28% ↓ mortality, espec if >80% of cases at center done radially (Lancet 2015;385:2465)

Periprocedural pharmacotherapy for PCI
- **Aspirin:** 325 mg × 1 (≥2 h prior to angio) → 81 mg qd
- **P2Y12 inhibitor** *(choose one):*
  clopidogrel: 600 mg × 1 → 75 mg qd; preRx ↓ MACE (JAMA 2005;294:1224 & 2012;308:2507)
  prasugrel or ticagrelor (only in ACS, qv)
  cangrelor (IV, short-acting): ↓ early ischemic events vs clopi given w/o preload (NEJM 2013;368:1303)
- **GP IIb/IIIa inhibitor:** *consider adding* abciximab, eptifibatide, or tirofiban; data showing ↓ MACE largely before routine P2Y12 inhibition and w/ UFH as anticoagulant. Remains reasonable espec if using clopidogrel and did not preRx.
- **Anticoagulant** *(choose one; typically d/c'd at end of PCI):*
  UFH: most common choice in U.S.
  bivalirudin: ↓ bleeding (espec vs UFH + GP IIb/IIIa inhib; JAMA 2015;313:1336), ± ↑ MI, ↑ stent thrombosis in STEMI (not mitigated by longer infusion), ↓ mortality in some but not all trials (Lancet 2014;384:599; MATRIX NEJM 2015); use if Pt has HIT
  enoxaparin (nb, cannot ✓ degree of anticoag)
- **Statin** (high-dose): PreRx ↓ peri-PCI myonecrosis (Circ 2011;123:1622) & ↓ risk of contrast-induced nephropathy (JACC 2014;63:71)

PCI options
- **Balloon angioplasty (POBA):** effective, but c/b dissection & elastic recoil & neointimal hyperplasia → restenosis; now reserved for small lesions & ? some SVG lesions
- **Bare metal stents (BMS):** ↓ elastic recoil → 33–50% ↓ restenosis & repeat revasc (to ~10% by 1 y) c/w POBA; requires P2Y12 inhibitor ≥4 weeks (ideally up to 6 mo)
- **Drug-eluting stents (DES)**
  antiproliferative drug released over several weeks → ↓ neointimal hyperplasia ~75% ↓ restenosis, ~50% ↓ repeat revasc (to <5% by 1 y), no Δ D/MI (NEJM 2013;368:254)
  delayed re-endothelialization & potentially proinflammatory polymers may cause ↑ in risk of late stent thrombosis; requires P2Y12 inhibitor ≥6 mo
  next generation DES (eg, w/ everolimus) w/ *lower* risk of stent thrombosis vs BMS (Lancet 2012;379:1393)

Other peri-PCI interventions
- **Fractional flow reserve (FFR):** ratio of max flow (induced by IV or IC adenosine) distal vs proximal to a stenosis; if used to guide PCI (ie, revasc only if FFR <0.8) → ↓ # stents & ↓ D/MI/revasc (NEJM 2009;360:213)
- **Thrombus aspiration:** small study showed manual aspiration of thrombus pre-PCI in STEMI ↓ mortality, but larger studies show no benefit and ↑ stroke (Lancet 2008;371:1915; NEJM 2013;369:1587 & 2015;372:1389)

Post-PCI complications
- Postprocedure ✓ vascular access site, distal pulses, ECG, CBC, Cr
- Vascular closure devices speed time to hemostasis and ↓ incidence of hematoma (JAMA 2014;312:1981)
- **Bleeding**
  hematoma/overt bleeding: **manual compression,** reverse/stop anticoag
  retroperitoneal bleed (if puncture above inguinal ligament)
  may p/w ↓ Hct ± flank or back pain; ↑ HR & ↓ BP late
  Dx w/ abd/pelvic CT (I−)
  Rx: reverse/stop anticoag (d/w interventionalist), IV fluids/PRBC/plts as required; if bleeding uncontrolled, consult performing interventionalist or surgery

- **Vascular damage** (~1% of dx angio, ~5% of PCI; *Circ* 2007;115:2666)
  pseudoaneurysm: hematoma w/ continued communication to artery
    can present w/ triad of pain, expansile mass, systolic bruit; diagnose w/ U/S;
    Rx (if *pain* or >2 cm): U/S-directed thrombin injection (>95% success, depends
      on anatomy); surgical repair if very large or if minimally invasive Rx fails
  AV fistula: continuous bruit; Dx: U/S; Rx: surgical repair
  limb ischemia (emboli, dissection, clot): cool, mottled extremity, ↓ distal pulses; Dx:
    pulse volume recording (PVR), angio; Rx: percutaneous or surgical repair
- **Peri-PCI MI:** >5× ULN of Tn/CK-MB + either sx or ECG/angio/imaging Δs; Qw MI in <1%
- **Renal failure:** contrast-induced manifests w/in 24 h, peaks 3–5 d (see "CIAKI")
- **Cholesterol emboli syndrome**
  typically seen in middle-aged & elderly and w/ heavy burden of aortic atheroma
  multiple clinical manifestations (although may be delay between cath & s/s) including:
    intact distal pulses but livedo reticularis pattern and toe necrosis ("blue toe syndrome")
    renal failure: late and progressive (thus unlike CIAKI), ± eos in urine
    mesenteric ischemia: abd pain, GIB, pancreatitis
    CNS: TIA, stroke, amaurosis fugax, Hollenhorst plaques (bright retinal lesion)
  Dx: can only be confirmed by biopsy; may see ↑ circulating eos, ↓ complement,
    ↑ CRP, ↑ ESR, ↑ plts, ↑ fibrinogen
  Rx: supportive; no clear benefit for anti-inflam or anticoagulant Rx
- **Stent thrombosis** (acute clot formation in stent): rare event, but high mortality
  can occur anytime between mins to yrs after PCI
  typically p/w ACS (often STEMI)
  typically due to either **mechanical problem** (stent underexpansion or unrecognized dissection, typically presents early) or **d/c of antiplt Rx** (espec if d/c both
    ASA & P2Y₁₂ inhib; *JAMA* 2005;293:2126)
- **In-stent restenosis** (neointimal hyperplasia): months after PCI, typically p/w gradual
  ↑ angina (10% p/w ACS). Due to combination of elastic recoil and neointimal
  hyperplasia; ↓ w/ DES vs BMS.

Duration of P2Y₁₂ inhibition
- In Pts w/ MI (qv), goal of antiplatelet therapy is ↓ CVD, MI, and stroke as well as
  rarer event of stent thrombosis. ∴ Long-term therapy *beyond* 12 mo is logical and
  has been shown to ↓ CV death, MI, and stroke (*NEJM* 2015;372:1791; *JACC* 2007;49:1982 &
  2015;65:2211).
- In Pts w/ SIHD, concern for late (>30 d) stent thrombosis led to recs for 12-mo
  duration, but newer generation stents have lower risk of stent thrombosis
- Several small trials showed shorter duration of P2Y₁₂ inhibition (3–6 vs 12 mo) led
  to nonstatistically significant higher rates of MI and ST (but still infrequent) but
  less bleeding (*JACC* 2012;60:1340; *JAMA* 2013;310:2510; *EHJ* 2015;36:1252)
- Much larger DAPT trial showed that longer inhibition (30 vs 12 mo) led to 29%
  ↓ MACE and 71% ↓ ST (although rates and absolute risk reduction very low with
  newer generation stents), but ↑ bleeding and, in Pts w/ SIHD, marginally significant
  ↑ mortality (driven by non-CV mortality) (*NEJM* 2014;371:2155)

Need for premature discontinuation of antiplatelet therapy
- If possible, postpone major invasive procedures ≥1 mo after BMS or ≥3–6 mo after DES
- If not possible and high of risk bleeding during procedure, d/c prasugrel 7 d, clopidogrel 5 d, or ticagrelor 5 d (per prescribing information, but in major clinical trial,
  just ~3 d prior to procedure. Continue ASA and resume P2Y₁₂ inhibitor w/ loading
  dose ASAP per surgery.
- If high-risk stent and bridging required, consider short-acting GP IIb/IIIa inhibitor (eptifibatide or tirofiban) from 3 d until 4–6 h prior to surgery (*Circ* 2013;128:2785). Consider
  cangrelor (IV reversible P2Y₁₂ inhib) (*JAMA* 2012;307:265).

Advances in CABG technique
- **"Mini-CABG"** = minimally invasive. Thoracotomy or partial sternotomy rather than
  full sternotomy. Advantages include ↓ pain & ↓ LOS. May be on- or off-pump.
- **Off-pump** ("beating heart surgery"): avoids cardiopulmonary bypass but makes
  anastomotic suturing more challenging. In 1 study, ↑ CV death and ↓ graft patency
  at 12 mo c/w on-pump (*NEJM* 2009;361:1827); other studies w/ ≈ mortality w/ off- vs
  on-pump.
- **Robotic:** type of mini-CABG where endoscopic instruments inserted via small incisions to anastomose the LIMA to the LAD on closed chest and beating heart
- **Hybrid procedures:** typically involves combo of LIMA-LAD mini-CABG with PCI
  of other vessels

ACUTE CORONARY SYNDROMES

Spectrum of Acute Coronary Syndromes			
Dx	**UA**	**NSTEMI**	**STEMI**
Coronary thrombosis	Subtotal occlusion		Total occlusion
History	angina that is new-onset, crescendo or at rest; usually <30 min		angina at rest
ECG	± ST depression and/or TWI		ST elevations
Troponin/CK-MB	⊖	⊕	⊕⊕

Ddx (causes of myocardial ischemia/infarction other than atherosclerotic plaque rupture)
- **Nonatherosclerotic coronary artery disease**
  Spasm: Prinzmetal's variant, cocaine-induced (6% of CP + cocaine use r/i for MI)
  Dissection: spontaneous (vasculitis, CTD, pregnancy), aortic dissection with retrograde extension (usually involving RCA → IMI) or mechanical (catheter, surgery, trauma)
  Embolism (Circ 2015;132:241): AF, thrombus/myxoma, endocard., prosth valve; thrombosis
  Vasculitis: Kawasaki syndrome, Takayasu arteritis, PAN, Churg-Strauss, SLE, RA
  Congenital: anomalous origin from aorta or PA (coronary compressed), myocardial bridge (intramural segment)
- **Ischemic imbalance not due to plaque rupture** ("type 2" MI): ↑ myocardial O_2 demand (eg, ↑ HR, anemia, AS) or ↓ supply (hypotension, severe anemia)
- **Direct myocardial injury:** myocarditis; Takotsubo/stress CMP; toxic CMP; cardiac contusion

Clinical manifestations (JAMA 2005;294:2623)
- **Typical angina:** retrosternal pressure/pain/tightness ± radiation to neck, jaw or arms precip. by exertion, relieved by rest or NTG; in ACS, new-onset, crescendo or at rest; see "Chest Pain" for likelihood ratios for different sx
- **Associated symptoms:** dyspnea, diaphoresis, N/V, palpitations or lightheadedness
- Many MIs (~20% in older series) are initially unrecognized b/c silent or atypical sx
- Atypical sxs (incl N/V & epig pain) may be more common with inferior ischemia
- Women may have ↑ freq of atypical sx vs men

Physical exam
- Signs of ischemia: S_4, new MR murmur 2° pap. muscle dysfxn, paradoxical S_2, diaphoresis
- Signs of heart failure: ↑ JVP, crackles in lung fields, ⊕ S_3, HoTN, cool extremities
- Signs of other vascular disease: asymmetric BP (aortic dissection or subclavian disease), carotid or femoral bruits, ↓ distal pulses

ECG
- ✓ w/in 10 min of presentation, q15–30min × 1 h if initial ECG non-dx, w/ any Δ in sx, and routinely at 6–12 h; compare w/ baseline
- Signs of ischemia (JAMA 1998;280:1256)
  STE: generally ≥1 mm in ≥2 contiguous leads (see "STEMI" for details)
  new or presumed new (ie, not known to be old) LBBB w/ compelling H&P
  STD ≥0.5 mm (⊕ LR 3–5), TWI ≥2 mm (⊕ LR 2–3), hyperacute Tw
- Qw or PRWP may suggest prior MI, ∴ higher pretest probability of CAD
- Dx of STEMI if old LBBB (Sgarbossa's criteria): ≥1 mm STE concordant w/ direction of QRS (Se 73%, Sp 92%), STD ≥1 mm V_1–V_3 (Se 25%, Sp 96%) or STE ≥5 mm discordant w/ QRS (Se 31%, Sp 92%)

Localization of MI		
Anatomic area	**ECG leads w/ STE**	**Coronary artery**
Septal	V_1–V_2	Proximal LAD
Anterior	V_3–V_4	LAD
Apical	V_5–V_6	Distal LAD, LCx or RCA
Lateral	I, aVL	LCx
Inferior	II, III, aVF	RCA (~85%), LCx (~15%)
RV	V_1–V_2 & V_4R (most Se)	Proximal RCA
Posterior	ST depression V_1–V_3 (= STE V_7–V_9 posterior leads)	RCA or LCx

If ECG non-dx and suspicion high, consider addt'l lateral (posterior) leads (V_7–V_9) to further assess distal LCx/ RCA territory. Check right-sided precordial leads in patients with IMI to help detect RV involvement (STE in V_4R most Se). STE in III > STE in II and lack of STE in I or aVL suggest RCA rather than LCx culprit in IMI.

Cardiac biomarkers
- Troponin (Tn) preferred over CK-MB
- ✓ Tn at baseline & 3–6 h after sx onset; may also ✓ beyond 6 h if high index of suspicion based on clinical presentation or ECGs or if sx Δ
- Rise to >99th %ile in approp. clinical setting dx of MI (see "Chest Pain")
- In Pts w/ ACS & ↓ CrCl, ↑ Tn still portends poor prognosis (*NEJM* 2002;346:2047)

Other potential dx tests
- If low prob, **stress test, CT angio** or rest perfusion imaging to r/o CAD (see "Chest Pain")
- TTE (new wall motion abnl) suggestive of ACS but not specific, as may be seen if old MI
- Coronary angio gold standard for evaluation of CAD

Prinzmetal's (variant) angina
- Coronary spasm → transient STE usually w/o MI (but MI, AVB, VT can occur)
- Pts usually young, smokers, ± other vasospastic disorders (eg, migraines, Raynaud's)
- Most frequent between midnight and early morning when vagal tone is highest
- Provocation testing: spasm can be precipitated at angio w/ IC ergonovine or acetylchol. positive test = severe narrowing w/ sx or ECG Δs; nonobstructive CAD typically seen; rarely done as risks include refractory/recurrent spasm or arrhythmia
- Noninvasive testing: hyperventilation, 12-lead Holter, exercise study
- Treatment: often initiated empirically without provocation testing:
  high-dose CCB (dilt, verap or nifed all roughly ≈) & standing nitrates (+SL prn)
  ? α-blockers/statins; d/c smoking
  avoid high-dose ASA (can inhibit prostacyclin & worsen spasm), nonselect βB, triptans
- Cocaine-induced vasospasm: use CCB, nitrates, ASA; ? avoid βB, but data weak and labetalol appears safe (*Archives* 2010;170:874; *Circ* 2011;123:2022)

Likelihood of ACS			
Feature	**High** (any of below)	**Intermediate** (no high features, any of below)	**Low** (no high/inter. features, may have below)
History	Chest or L arm pain like prior angina, h/o CAD (incl MI)	Chest or arm pain age >70 y, male, diabetes	Atypical sx (eg, pleuritic, sharp or positional pain)
Exam	HoTN, diaphoresis, HF, transient MR	PAD or cerebrovascular dis.	Pain reproduced on palp.
ECG	New STD (≥1 mm) TWI in mult leads	Old Qw, STD (0.5–0.9 mm), TWI (>1 mm)	TWF/TWI (<1 mm) in leads w/ dominant R wave
Biomarkers	⊕ Tn or CK-MB	Normal	Normal

(Adapted from ACC/AHA 2007 Guideline Update for UA/NSTEMI, *Circ* 2007;116:e148)

Approach to triage
- If hx and initial ECG & Tn non-dx, repeat ECG q15–30min × 1 h & Tn 3–6 h after sx onset
- If remain nl and low likelihood of ACS, search for alternative causes of chest pain
- If remain nl, have ruled out MI, *but* if suspicion for ACS based on hx, then still need to r/o UA w/ stress test to assess for inducible ischemia (or CTA to r/o CAD);
  if low risk (eg, age ≤70; ø prior CAD, CVD, PAD; ø rest angina) can do before d/c from ED or as outPt w/in 72 h (0% mortality, <0.5% MI, *Ann Emerg Med* 2006;47:427)
  if not low risk, admit and initiate Rx for possible ACS and consider stress test or cath

Acute Anti-Ischemic and Analgesic Treatment	
Nitrates (SL or IV) 0.3–0.4 mg SL q5min ×3, then consider IV if still sx	Use for relief of sx, control HTN or Rx of HF No clear ↓ in mortality *Caution* if preload-sensitive (eg, HoTN, AS, sx RV infarct); contraindic if recent PDE5 inhibit use
β-blockers eg, metop 25–50 mg PO q6h titrate slowly to HR 50–60 IV only if HTN and no HF	↓ ischemia & progression of UA to MI (*JAMA* 1988;260:2259) STEMI: ~20% ↓ arrhythmic death or reMI, but 30% ↑ cardiogenic shock early (espec if signs of HF), & ∴ no Δ overall mortality (*Lancet* 2005;366:1622) In Pts w/o HF, IV βB prior to 1° PCI ↓ infarct size and ↑ EF (*Circ* 2013;128:1495) *Contraindic.* PR >0.24 sec, HR <60, 2°/3° AVB, severe bronchospasm, s/s HF or low output, risk factors for shock (eg, >70 y, HR >110, SBP <120, late presentation STEMI)
CCB (nondihydropyridines)	If cannot tolerate βB b/c bronchospasm; otherwise has similar contraindications as βB Rx

Morphine	Relieves pain, ↓ anxiety, venodilation → ↓ preload ∴ use for persistent sx or CHF. Do not mask refractory sx. May delay onset of antiplatelet Rx (JACC 2014;63:630)
Oxygen	Use prn for resp distress or to keep S_aO₂ >90% ? ↑ infarct size in STEMI w/o hypoxia (Circ 2015;131:2143)

Other early adjunctive therapy
- **High-intensity statin therapy** (eg, atorvastatin 80 mg qd)
  ↓ ischemic events w/ benefit emerging w/in wks (JAMA 2001;285:1711 & JACC 2005;46:1405)
  ↓ peri-PCI MI (JACC 2010;56:1099); ↓ contrast-induced nephropathy (JACC 2014;63:71)
- **ACEI/ARB:** start once hemodynamics and renal function stable
  Strong indication for ACEI if heart failure, EF <40%, HTN, DM, CKD; ~10% ↓ mortality,
  greatest benefit in ant. STEMI or prior MI (Lancet 1994;343:1115 & 1995;345:669)
  Start w/ low dose of short-acting (eg, captopril 6.25 mg tid), titrate up as tolerated
  ARB appear ≈ ACEI (NEJM 2003;349:20); if used if contraindic to ACEI
- Ezetimibe, aldosterone blockade, and ranolazine discussed later (long-term Rx)
- **IABP:** can be used for refractory angina when PCI not available

NSTE-ACS (Circ 2014;130:e344)

Key issues are antithrombotic regimen and invasive vs conservative strategy

Antiplatelet Therapy	
Aspirin 162–325 mg × 1, then 81 mg qd (non-enteric coated, chewable)	50–70% ↓ D/MI (NEJM 1988;319:1105) Low dose (~81 mg) pref long term (NEJM 2010;363:930) If allergy, use clopi and/or desensitize to ASA
P2Y₁₂ (ADP receptor) inhibitor (choose one of the following in addition to ASA). Timing remains controversial. Some data support benefit of clopidogrel preRx prior to angiography (JAMA 2012;308:2507). Ticagrelor was given upstream in pivotal study. Prasugrel should be given once PCI planned (ie, anatomy defined). European guidelines recommend P2Y₁₂ inhibitor as soon as possible after presentation (EHJ 2011;32:2999).	
• **Ticagrelor** 180 mg × 1 → 90 mg bid Reversible binding, but wait 3–5 d prior to surg Use only with ASA <100 mg qd	Preferred over clopidogrel More rapid and potent plt inhib c/w clopi 16% ↓ CVD/MI/stroke & 21% ↓ CV death c/w clopi; ↑ non-CABG bleeding (NEJM 2009;361:1045) Sensation of dyspnea (S_aO₂ & PFTs nl) and ventricu- lar pauses; perhaps b/c blocks adenosine reuptake
• **Prasugrel** 60 mg × 1 at PCI → 10 mg qd (consider 5 mg/d if <60 kg) Wait 7 d prior to surgery	Use at time of PCI; preferred over clopidogrel More rapid and potent plt inhib c/w clopi 19% ↓ CVD/MI/stroke in ACS w/ planned PCI vs clopi, but ↑ bleeding (NEJM 2007;359:2001), incl fatal bleeds Not sup to clopi if med mgmt w/o PCI (NEJM 2012;367:1297) In NSTE-ACS, should be given at time of PCI and not upstream due to ↑ bleeding (NEJM 2013;369:999) Contraindic. if h/o TIA/CVA; ? avoid if >75 y
• **Clopidogrel*** 300–600 mg × 1 → 75 mg qd Requires ~6 h to steady state	ASA+clopi ≈ 20% ↓ CVD/MI/stroke vs ASA alone ↑ benefit if given hrs prior to PCI, but then if require CABG, need to wait >5 d after d/c clopi
• **Cangrelor** Only IV P2Y₁₂ inhibitor Rapid onset/offset; t½ 3–5 min	22% ↓ CV events (mostly peri-PCI MI and stent thrombosis) vs clopi 300 mg at time of PCI; no significant ↑ bleeding (NEJM 2013;368:1303) Unclear benefit if upstream clopi (NEJM 2009;361:2318) and no data vs prasugrel or ticagrelor
GP IIb/IIIa inhibitors (GPI) Abciximab: LD 0.25 mg/kg IV, then 0.125 mcg/kg/min Eptifibatide: LD 180 mcg/kg IV ×2, then 2 mcg/kg/min (½ dose if CrCl <50 mL/min) Tirofiban: LD 25 mcg/kg IV, then 0.15 mcg/kg/min (½ dose if CrCl <30 mL/min)	No clear benefit for routinely starting prior to PCI and ↑ bleeding (NEJM 2009;360:2176). Consider epti or tiro if refractory ischemia despite optimal Rx while awaiting angio. Consider in high-risk Pts (eg, large thrombus burden) at time of PCI, espec if using clopi and not preRx'd. Often administered 18–24 h post PCI, but shorter duration (~2 h) may be as efficacious and with ↓ bleeding (JACC 2009;53:837); D/C eptifibatide/tirofiban ≥2–4 h and abciximab ≥12 h prior to urgent CABG.

*Utility of platelet function testing remains unproven (JAMA 2011;305:1097; NEJM 2012;367:2100), but studies underpowered. ~30% pop has ↓ fxn CYP2C19 allele → ↑ CV events if PCI on clopi compared w/ wild type (NEJM 2009;360:354; JAMA 2010;304:1821).

Anticoagulant Therapy (choose one)	
UFH: 60 U/kg IVB (max 4000 U) then 12 U/kg/h (max 1000 U/h initially) × 48 h or until end of PCI	24% ↓ D/MI (*JAMA* 1996;276:811) Titrate to aPTT 1.5–2× control (~50–70 sec) Hold until INR <2 if already on warfarin
Enoxaparin (low-molec-wt heparin) 1 mg/kg SC bid (± 30 mg IVB) (qd if CrCl <30) × 2–8 d or until PCI	~10% ↓ D/MI vs UFH (*JAMA* 2004;292:45,89). Can perform PCI on enox (*Circ* 2001;103:658), but ↑ bleeding if switch b/w enox and UFH.
Bivalirudin (direct thrombin inhibitor) 0.75 mg/kg IVB at PCI → 1.75 mg/kg/h	↓ bleeding (espec vs UFH + GPI), ± ↑ early MI (*Lancet* 2014;384:599). Use instead of UFH if HIT.
Fondaparinux (Xa inhibitor) 2.5 mg SC qd × 2–8 d	C/w enox, 17% ↓ death & 38% ↓ bleeding (*NEJM* 2006;354:1464). However, ↑ risk of catheter thrombosis; ∴ must supplement w/ UFH if PCI.

Coronary angiography (*Circ* 2014;130:e344)
- **Immediate/urgent coronary angiography** (w/in 2 h) if refractory/recurrent angina or hemodynamic or electrical instability
- **Invasive (INV) strategy** = routine angiography w/in 72 h (*NEJM* 2009;360:2165)
  Early (w/in 24 h) if: ⊕ Tn, ST Δ, GRACE risk score (www.outcomes-umassmed.org/grace) >140
  Delayed (ie, acceptable anytime w/in 72 h) if no indication for early/immediate cath but has other high-risk predictors incl: diabetes, EF <40%, GFR <60, post-MI angina, TIMI Risk Score ≥3, GRACE score 109–140, PCI w/in 6 mo, prior CABG
  Invasive strategy leads to 32% ↓ rehosp for ACS, nonsignif 16% ↓ MI, no Δ in mortality c/w cons. (*JAMA* 2008;300:71); ↑ peri-PCI MI counterbalanced by ↓↓ in spont. MI; mortality benefit seen in some studies, likely only if cons. strategy w/ low rate of angio ↑ risk of death or MI if invasive strategy deferred beyond 72 h (*JAMA* 2003;290:1593)
- **Conservative (CONS) strategy** = selective angio. Medical Rx with pre-d/c stress test; angio only if recurrent ischemia or ⊕ ETT. Indicated for: low TIMI Risk Score, Pt or physician preference in absence of high-risk features, low-risk women (*JAMA* 2008;300:71).

TIMI Risk Score (TRS) for UA/NSTEMI (*JAMA* 2000;284:835)				
Calculation of Risk Score			**Application of Risk Score**	
Characteristic	**Point**		**Score**	**D/MI/UR by 14 d**
Historical			0–1	5%
Age ≥65 y	1		2	8%
≥3 Risk factors for CAD	1		3	13%
Known CAD (stenosis ≥50%)	1		4	20%
ASA use in past 7 d	1		5	26%
Presentation			6–7	41%
Severe angina (≥2 episodes w/in 24 h)	1		Higher risk Pts (TRS ≥3) derive ↑ benefit from LMWH, GP IIb/IIIa inhibitors and early angiography (*JACC* 2003;41:89S)	
ST deviation ≥0.5 mm	1			
⊕ cardiac marker (troponin, CK-MB)	1			
RISK SCORE = Total points	**(0–7)**			

Figure 1-2 Approach to UA/NSTEMI

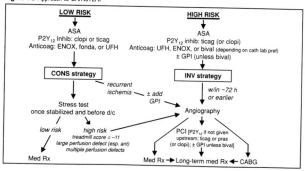

STEMI

Requisite STE (at J point)
- ≥2 contiguous leads w/ ≥1 mm (except for V_2–V_3: ≥2 mm in ♂ and ≥1.5 mm in ♀), or
- New or presumed new LBBB w/ compelling H&P, or
- True posterior MI: ST depression V_1–V_3 + tall Rw w/ STE on posterior leads (V_7–V_9)

Reperfusion ("time is muscle")
- Immediate reperfusion (ie, opening occluded culprit coronary artery) is critical
- In PCI-capable hospital, goal should be **primary PCI w/in 90 min** of 1st medical contact
- In non–PCI-capable hospital, consider *transfer* to PCI-capable hospital (see below), o/w fibrinolytic therapy w/in 30 min of hospital presentation. If dx confirmed, administration of fibrinolytic in ambulance prior to arrival can be considered
- Do not let decision regarding *method* of reperfusion delay *time* to reperfusion

Primary PCI (NEJM 2007;356:47; JACC 2013;61:e78)
- Definition: immediate PCI upon arrival to hospital or transfer for immediate PCI
- Indications: STE + sx onset <12 h; ongoing ischemia 12–24 h after sx onset; shock or severe HF regardless of time
- Superior to lysis: 27% ↓ death, 65% ↓ reMI, 54% ↓ stroke, 95% ↓ ICH (Lancet 2003;361:13)
- *Transfer* to center for 1° PCI superior to lysis (NEJM 2003;349:733). ∴ If initially seen at non-PCI capable hosp, transfer for PCI if door-in to door-out time can be ≤30 min and 1st medical contact to PCI time estimated to be ≤120 min.
- Thrombus aspiration: small study showed ↓ mortality, but larger studies show no benefit and ↑ stroke (Lancet 2008;371:1915; NEJM 2013;369:1587 & 2015;372:1389)
- Small studies have demonstrated ↓ MACE w/ complete revasc vs culprit artery alone (NEJM 2013; 369:1115; JACC 2015;65:963), large study ongoing; alternatively, could assess ischemia due to residual lesions w/ imaging stress (Circ 2011;124:e574)

Fibrinolysis vs Hospital Transfer for Primary PCI: Assess Time and Risk
1. **Time required for transport to skilled PCI lab**: door-to-balloon <120 min & [door-to-balloon]–[door-to-needle] <1 h favors transfer for PCI
2. **Risk from STEMI**: high-risk Pts (eg, shock) fare better with mechanical reperfusion
3. **Time to presentation**: efficacy of lytics ↓ w/ ↑ time from sx onset, espec >3 h
4. **Risk of fibrinolysis**: if high risk of ICH or bleeding, PCI safer option

Adapted from ACC/AHA 2013 STEMI Guidelines (Circ 2013;127:529)

Fibrinolysis
- Indic: STE/LBBB + sx <12 h + >120 min before PCI can be performed; benefit if sx >12 h less clear; reasonable if persist. sx & STE or hemodyn instability or large territory at risk
- Fibrin-spec lytics (TNK, TPA, RPA) ↑ artery patency vs streptokinase (JACC 2013;61:e78)
- Mortality ↓ ~20% in anterior MI or LBBB and ~10% in IMI c/w ∅ reperfusion Rx
- Prehospital lysis (ie, ambulance): further 17% ↓ in mortality (JAMA 2000;283:2686)
- ~1% risk of ICH; high-risk groups include elderly (~2% if >75 y), women, low wt
- Although age not contraindic., ↑ risk of ICH in elderly (>75 y) makes PCI more attractive
- Successful reperfusion gauged by sx & ECG: sudden CP resolution & ≥70% resolution of STE indicative of successful reperfusion; conversely, STE resolution <50% after 60–90 min should prompt consideration of rescue PCI (qv)

Contraindications to Fibrinolysis	
Absolute contraindications	**Relative contraindications**
• Any prior ICH	• Hx of severe HTN or SBP >180 or DBP >110 on presentation (? absolute contra. if low-risk MI)
• Intracranial neoplasm, aneurysm, AVM	
• Ischemic stroke w/in 3 mo (unless acute w/in 4.5 h) or closed head trauma w/in 3 mo	• Ischemic stroke >3 mo prior
	• Dementia
	• Recent traumatic or prolonged CPR >10 min
• Active internal bleeding or known bleeding diathesis	• Trauma or major surgery w/in 3 wk
• Head/facial trauma w/in 3 mo	• Recent internal bleed (w/in 2–4 wk); active PUD
• Head/spinal surgery w/in 2 mo	• Noncompressible vascular punctures
• Suspected aortic dissection	• Prior SK exposure (if considering SK)
• Severe uncontrollable HTN	• Pregnancy
• For SK, SK Rx w/in 6 mo	• Current use of anticoagulants

Nonprimary PCI

- Facilitated or pharmacoinvasive PCI = upstream lytic, GPI or GPI + ½ dose lytic before PCI; in general no clear clinical benefit & ↑ bleeding (Lancet 2006;367:569; NEJM 2013;368:1379)
- Rescue PCI if shock, unstable, failed reperfusion or persistent sx (NEJM 2005;353:2758)
- Routine angio ± PCI w/in 24 h of successful lysis: ↓ D/MI/revasc (Lancet 2004;364:1045) and w/in 6 h ↓ reMI, recurrent ischemia, & HF compared to w/in 2 wk (NEJM 2009;360:2705); ∴ if lysed at non-PCI capable hospital, consider transfer to PCI-capable hospital ASAP espec if high-risk presentation (eg, anterior MI, inferior MI w/ low EF or RV infarct, extensive STE or LBBB, HF, ↓ BP or ↑ HR)
- Late PCI (median day 8) of occluded infarct-related artery: no benefit (NEJM 2006;355:2395)

Antiplatelet Therapy	
Aspirin 162–325 mg × 1 (crushed/chewed) then 81 mg qd	23% ↓ in death (Lancet 1988;ii:349) Should not be stopped if CABG required
P2Y₁₂ inhibitor Give ASAP (do not wait for angio) Ticagrelor or prasugrel (if PCI as detailed above) Clopidogrel: 600 mg pre-PCI; 300 mg if lysis (no LD if >75 y) → 75 mg qd	Lysis: clopidogrel 41% ↑ in patency, 7% ↓ mort, no Δ major bleed or ICH (NEJM 2005;352:1179; Lancet 2005;366:1607); no data for pras or ticag w/ lytic PCI: prasugrel and ticagrelor ↓ CV events c/w clopi (Lancet 2009;373:723 & Circ 2010;122:2131) Nb, antiplt effects delayed in STEMI Pts
GP IIb/IIIa inhibitors abciximab, eptifibatide, tirofiban	Lysis: no indication (Lancet 2001;357:1905) Peri-PCI: 60% ↓ D/MI/UR (NEJM 2001;344:1895)

Adapted from ACC/AHA 2013 STEMI Guidelines Update (Circ 2013;127:529); Lancet 2013;382:633

Anticoagulant Therapy (choose one)	
UFH 60 U/kg IVB (max 4000 U) 12 U/kg/h (max 1000 U/h initially)	No demonstrated mortality benefit ↑ patency with fibrin-specific lytics Titrate to aPTT 1.5–2× control (~50–70 sec)
Enoxaparin Lysis: 30 mg IVB → 1 mg/kg SC bid (adjust for age >75 & CrCl) PCI: 0.5 mg/kg IVB	Lysis: 17% ↓ D/MI w/ ENOX × 7 d vs UFH × 2 d (NEJM 2006;354:1477) PCI: ↓ D/MI/revasc and ≈ bleeding vs UFH (Lancet 2011;378:693)
Bivalirudin 0.75 mg/kg IVB → 1.75 mg/kg/hr IV (ongoing research on prolonged infusions)	PCI: ↓ bleeding (espec vs UFH + GP IIb/IIIa inhib), ± ↑ MI, ↑ stent thromb (not mitigated by longer infusion), ↓ mortality in some but not all trials (Lancet 2014;384:599; JAMA 2015;313:1336; MATRIX NEJM 2015)
Fondaparinux 2.5 mg IVB → 2.5 mg SC qd Contraindic if CrCl ≤30 mL/min	Lysis: superior to placebo & to UFH, with less bleeding (JAMA 2006;295:1519) PCI: risk of catheter thromb.; should not be used

Adapted from ACC/AHA 2013 STEMI Guidelines Update (Circ 2013;127:529); Lancet 2013;382:633

Intraaortic Balloon Pump (IABP) Counterpulsation

- Inflates during diastole and deflates during systole to ↑ coronary flow and ↓ afterload
- Routine use in high-risk STEMI → ↑ stroke/bleeds w/o Δ in survival, infarct size or EF (EHJ 2009;30:459; JAMA 2011;306:1329)
- In cardiogenic shock, no survival benefit w/ IABP if early revasc (NEJM 2012;367:1287); 18% ↓ death in Pts w/ cardiogenic shock treated with lytic (EHJ 2009;30:459)

LV failure (~25%)

- Diurese to achieve PCWP 15–20 → ↓ pulmonary edema, ↓ myocardial O₂ demand
- ↓ Afterload → ↑ stroke volume & CO, ↓ myocardial O₂ demand can use IV NTG or nitroprusside (risk of coronary steal) → short-acting ACEI
- Inotropes if HF despite diuresis & ↓ afterload; use dopamine, dobutamine or milrinone
- **Cardiogenic shock** (~7%): MAP <60 mmHg, CI <2 L/min/m², PCWP >18 mmHg; inotropes, mech support [eg, VAD, IABP (see above)] to keep CI >2; pressors to keep MAP >60; if not done already, coronary revasc (NEJM 1999;341:625)

IMI complications (Circ 1990;81:401; NEJM 1994;330:1211; JACC 2003;41:1273)

- **Heart block** (~20%, occurs because RCA typically supplies AV node) 40% on present., 20% w/in 24 h, rest by 72 h; high-grade AVB can develop abruptly Rx: atropine, epi, aminophylline (100 mg min × 2.5 min), temp pacing wire
- **RV infarct** (proximal RCA occlusion → compromised flow to RV marginal branch) Angiographically in 30–50%, but only ½ of those clinically signif. HoTN; ↑ JVP, ⊕ Kussmaul's; 1 mm STE in V₄R; RA/PCWP ≥0.8; RV dysfxn on TTE

Rx: optimize preload (RA goal 10–14, *BHJ* 1990;63:98); ↑ contractility (dobutamine); maintain AV synchrony (pacing as necessary); reperfusion (*NEJM* 1998;338:933); mechanical support (IABP or RVAD); pulmonary vasodilators (eg, inhaled NO)

Mechanical complications (incid. <1% for each; typically occur a few days post-MI)
- **Free wall rupture:** ↑ risk w/ lysis, large MI, ↑ age, ♀, HTN; p/w PEA or hypoTN, pericardial sx, tamponade; Rx: volume resusc., ? pericardiocentesis, inotropes, **surgery**
- **VSD:** large MI, esp in elderly; AMI → apical VSD, IMI → basal septum; 90% w/ harsh murmur ± thrill (*NEJM* 2002;347:1426); Rx: diuretics, vasodil., inotropes, IABP, **surgery**, perc. closure
- **Papillary muscle rupture:** more common after inf MI (PM pap. muscle supplied by PDA alone) than ant MI (AL pap. muscle supplied by diags & OMs); 50% w/ new murmur, rarely a thrill, ↑ v wave in PCWP tracing; asymmetric pulmonary edema on CXR (often worse in RUL due to direction of jet). Rx: diuretics, vasodilators, IABP, **surgery.**

Arrhythmias post-MI
- Treat as per ACLS for unstable or symptomatic bradycardias & tachycardias
- **AF** (10–16% incidence); βB or amio, ± digoxin (particularly if HF), heparin
- **VT/VF:** lido or amio × 6–24 h, then reassess; ↑ βB as tol., replete K & Mg, r/o ischemia; early monomorphic (<48 h post-MI) does *not* carry bad prognosis. Beyond 48 h, VT/VF a/w worse prognosis → consider wearable defibrillator (qv).
- Accelerated idioventricular rhythm (AIVR): slow VT (<100 bpm), often seen after successful reperfusion; typically self-terminates and does not require treatment
- May consider **backup transcutaneous pacing** (TP) if: 2° AVB type I, BBB
- **Backup TP or initiate transvenous pacing** if: 2° AVB type II; BBB + AVB
- **Transvenous pacing (TV)** if: 3° AVB; new BBB + 2° AVB type II; alternating LBBB/RBBB (can bridge w/ TP until TV, which is best accomplished under fluoroscopic guidance)

Other Post-MI Complications		
Complication	Clinical features	Treatment
LV thrombus	~30% incid. (espec lg antero-apical MI)	Anticoagulate × 3–6 mo
Ventricular aneurysm	Noncontractile outpouching of LV; 8 15% incid. (espec ant); persist STE	Surgery or perc repair if HF, thromboemboli, arrhythmia
Ventricular pseudoaneurysm	Rupture → sealed by thrombus and pericardium (espec in inf). Typically w/ narrow neck as c/w true aneurysm; Dx w/ cardiac MRI, CTA, or TEE.	Urgent surgery (or percutaneous repair)
Pericarditis	10–20% incid.; 1–4 d post-MI ⓘ pericardial rub; ECG Δs rare	High-dose ASA > aceta., colchicine, narcotics; minimize anticoag
Dressler's syndrome	<4% incid.; 2–10 wk post-MI fever, pericarditis, pleuritis	High-dose aspirin, NSAIDs

Prognosis
- In registries, in-hospital mortality is 6% w/ reperfusion Rx (lytic or PCI) and ~20% w/o
- Predictors of mortality: age, time to Rx, anterior MI or LBBB, heart failure (*Circ* 2000;102:2031)

Killip Class		
Class	Definition	Mort.
I	no CHF	6%
II	⊕ S₃ and/or basilar rales	17%
III	pulmonary edema	30–40%
IV	cardiogenic shock	60–80%

(*Am J Cardiol* 1967;20:457)

Forrester Class Mortality			
		PCWP (mmHg)	
		<18	>18
CI	>2.2	3%	9%
	≤2.2	23%	51%

(*NEJM* 1976;295:1356)

TIMI Risk Score for STEMI					
Characteristic	Points	Characteristic (cont)	Points	Score	30-d death
Age 65–74/≥75 y	2/3	Ant MI or new LBBB	1	0–2	~1–2%
SBP <100 mmHg	3	h/o DM, HTN or angina	1	3–4	~4–6%
HR >100 bpm	2	Wt <67 kg	1	5–6	~10–15%
Killip class II-IV	2	Time to Rx >4 h	1	≥7	≥20%

(*JAMA* 2001;286:1356)

Risk stratification
* Stress test if anatomy undefined; consider stress if signif residual CAD post-PCI of culprit
* Assess LVEF prior to d/c; EF ↑ ~6% in STEMI over 6 mo (*JACC* 2007;50:149)

Medications (barring contraindications)
* **Aspirin:** 81 mg daily
* **P2Y$_{12}$ inhib** (ticagrelor or prasugrel preferred over clopi): treat for *at least* 12 mo
    Prolonged Rx beyond 12 mo → ↓ CV death, MI, & stroke (& stent thrombosis) w/
    ↑ in bleeding, but no ↓ fatal bleeding or ICH. For Rx beyond 1st 12 mo, compa-
    rable efficacy w/ ticagrelor 90 or 60 mg bid, better safety & tolerability with 60 bid
    (*NEJM* 2015;372:1791; *JACC* 2007;49:1982 & 2015;65:2211).
    Some PPIs interfere w/ biotransformation of clopi and ∴ plt inhibition, but no
    convincing impact on clinical outcomes (*Lancet* 2009;374:989; *NEJM* 2010;363:1909); use
    w/PPIs if h/o GIB or multiple GIB risk factors (*JACC* 2010;56:2051)
* **β-blocker:** 23% ↓ mortality after MI
* **Statin:** high-intensity lipid-lowering (eg, atorvastatin 80 mg, *NEJM* 2004;350:1495)
* **Ezetimibe:** ↓ CV events including MI and ischemic stroke when added to statin
    (IMPROVE-IT, *NEJM* 2015;372:1500)
* **ACEI:** lifelong if HF, ↓ EF, HTN, DM; 4–6 wk or at least until hosp. d/c in all STEMI
    ? long-term benefit in CAD w/o HF (*NEJM* 2000;342:145 & 2004;351:2058; *Lancet* 2003;362:782)
* **Aldosterone antag:** 15% ↓ mortality if EF <40% & either s/s of HF or DM; contra-
    indic if renal dysfxn (Cr >2.5 in men, >2 in women) or K >5 (*NEJM* 2003;348:1309)
* **Nitrates:** standing if symptomatic; SL NTG prn for all
* **Ranolazine:** inhibits late inward Na current, prevents intracellular Ca overload;
    ↓ recurrent ischemia (*JAMA* 2007;297:1775)
* **Oral anticoagulants:** if warfarin needed in addition to ASA/clopi (eg, AF or LV throm-
    bus), target INR 2–2.5. ? stop ASA if at high bleeding risk on triple Rx (*Lancet*
    2013;381:1107). Not FDA approved: low-dose rivaroxaban (2.5 mg bid) in addition to
    ASA & clopi → 16% ↓ D/MI/stroke and 32% ↓ all-cause death, but ↑ major bleeding
    and ICH (*NEJM* 2012;366:9).
* **NSAIDs/COX2 inhib** relatively contraindic b/c ? ↑ death, MI, HF, rupture (*Circ* 2006;113:2906)

ICD (*NEJM* 2008;359:2245)
* If sust. VT/VF >2 d post-MI not due to reversible ischemia; consider wearable defibril-
    lator or ICD (*JACC* 2014;130:94)
* Indicated in 1° prevention of SCD if post-MI w/ EF ≤30–40% (NYHA II–III) or ≤30–35%
    (NYHA I); need to wait ≥40 d after MI (*NEJM* 2004;351:2481 & 2009;361:1427)

Risk factors and lifestyle modifications (*Circ* 2014;129(Suppl 2):S1 & S76)
* Low chol. (<200 mg/d) & fat (<7% saturated) diet; ? Ω-3 FA
* Traditional LDL-C goal <70 mg/dL; new recs w/o LDL-C target, rather simply high-
    intensity statin; may change w/ IMPROVE-IT trial showing that lower is better
    (lower CV event rate in arm with achieved LDL-C of 54 vs 70 mg/dL)
* BP <140/90 and consider <130/80 mmHg (*HTN* 2015;65:1372); smoking cessation
* If diabetic, tailor HbA1c goal based on Pt (avoid TZDs if HF)
* Exercise (30–60 min 5–7×/wk); cardiac rehab; BMI goal 18.5–24.9 kg/m^2
* Influenza & pneumococcal vaccination (*Circ* 2006;114:1549; *JAMA* 2013;310:1711); screen for
    depression

CARDIAC RISK ASSESSMENT FOR NONCARDIAC SURGERY

Goal: characterize risk of Pt & procedure → appropriate testing (ie, results will Δ management) and interventions (ie, reasonable probability of ↓ risk of MACE)

Preoperative assessment
- Clinical assessment: evidence of active cardiac disease and/or risk factors
- Functional capacity (METs)
- Surgery-specific risk

Clinical Assessment	
Active cardiac conditions	**Clinical risk factors**
• MI w/in 30 d or current unstable or severe angina • Decompensated HF • Significant arrhythmia (eg, Mobitz II, high-grade AVB, 3° AVB, new or sx VT, SVT w/ HR >100, sx brady) • Severe AS or sx MS	• h/o ischemic heart disease • h/o congestive HF • h/o stroke or TIA • Diabetes on insulin • Renal insuffic. (Cr >2 mg/dL)

Functional Capacity		
1–4 METs (poor)	**4–10 METs (moderate-to-good)**	**>10 METs (excellent)**
• ADLs • Walk indoors • Walk 1–2 level blocks	• Climb a flight of stairs/hill • Walk briskly; heavy housework • Golf, doubles tennis	• Strenuous sports

Surgery-Specific Risk		
High (>5% risk)	**Intermediate (1–5%)**	**Low (<1%)**
• Aortic or other major vascular • Peripheral vasc.	• Intrathoracic; intraperitoneal; prostate & major urologic • CEA; head & neck • Orthopedic	• Endoscopic • Breast; superficial • Cataract; ambulatory • Dental

Noninvasive Testing Result		
High risk	**Intermediate risk**	**Low risk**
Ischemia at <4 METs manifested by ≥1 of: • Horiz/down ST ↓ ≥1 mm or STE • ≥5 abnl leads or ischemic ECG Δs lasting >3 min after exertion • SBP ↓ 10 mmHg or typical angina	*Ischemia at 4–6 METs manifested by ≥1 of:* • Horiz/down ST ↓ ≥1 mm • 3–4 abnl leads • 1–3 min after exertion	No ischemia or at >7 METs w/ • ST ↓ ≥1 mm or • 1–2 abnl leads
Imaging with excellent NPV, poor PPV. Consider if high-risk patient.		

- **Revised Cardiac Risk Index (RCRI):** 6 risk factors = 5 clinical risk factors above and type of surgery (intrathoracic, intra-abd, or suprainguinal vascular) *(Circ 1999;100:1043)*
  # of risk factors predicts risk of MACE: ≤1 RF → <1%, 2 RFs → 6.6%, ≥3 RFs → 11%
- Comorbidity indices (eg, Charlson index) may predict mortality *(Am J Med Qual 2011;26:461)*

Preoperative testing *(Circ 2014;130:e278)*
- ECG if known cardiac disease and possibly reasonable in all, except if low-risk surgery
- TTE if any of the following and prior TTE >12 mo ago or prior to Δ in sx:
  dyspnea of unknown origin
  hx of HF w/ ↑ dyspnea
  suspected valvular disease (eg, murmur on exam)
  ≥moderate stenosis/regurg
- Stress test (usually pharmacologic) if:
  active cardiac issues where stress testing is indicated (qv), or
  not low-risk surgery, RCRI ≥2, poor or unknown fxnal capacity, and results *will Δ mgmt* (ie, modify or delay surgery, undergo coronary revascularization, etc.)
  overall low PPV to predict periop CV events
- Angiography: based on noninvasive stress results for standard indications, although systematic angio ↓ 2–5 y mortality in Pts undergoing vascular surgery *(JACC 2009;54:989)*
- ? consider CXR & ECG in preop evaluation of severely obese Pts *(Circ 2009;120:86)*

Coronary artery disease
- If possible, wait ~60 d after MI in the absence of revascularization before elective surgery
- After PCI: delay elective surgery 14 d after balloon angioplasty, 30 d after BMS implantation, and ideally 6 mo after DES implantation

- Coronary revascularization should be based on standard indications (eg, ACS, refractory sx, lg territory at risk). Has not been shown to Δ risk of death or postop MI when done prior to elective vasc. surgery based on perceived cardiac risk (*NEJM* 2004;351:2795) or documented extensive ischemia (*AJC* 2009;103:897).

Heart failure
- Decompensated HF should be optimally treated prior to elective surgery
- ↓ EF (<30%) associated with poor outcomes
- 30-d CV event rate: symptomatic HF > asx HFrEF > asx HFpEF > no HF

Valvular heart disease
- If meet criteria for valve intervention (qv), do so before elective surgery (postpone if necessary)
- If severe valve disease and surgery urgent, intra- & postoperative hemodynamic monitoring reasonable (espec for AS, since as ↑ risk even if sx not severe; be careful to maintain preload, avoid hypotension, and watch for atrial fibrillation)
- If severe AS and Pt not eligible for or impractical to do AVR prior to noncardiac surgery, balloon aortic valvuloplasty (BAV) and transcatheter aortic valve replacement (TAVR) can be considered but not routinely recommended (*Circ* 2008;118:e523)

Cardiac implantable electronic devices (CIEDs)
- Includes PPM, CRT, ICD
- Should be discussion between surgical team & CIED team regarding:
  - need for device (eg, complete heart block) & consequences if interference w/ fxn
  - likelihood of electromagnetic interference
  - consideration of reprogramming, magnet use, etc.

Pre- & perioperative pharmacologic management
- **ASA:** continue in Pts w/ existing indication. Initiation just prior to surgery does not ↓ 30-d ischemic events and ↑ bleeding (*NEJM* 2014;370:1494), but Pts w/ recent stents excluded.
- **Dual antiplatelet therapy** in Pts undergoing urgent surgery: continue 4–6 wk after PCI (BMS or DES) unless risk of bleeding > benefit of prevention of stent thrombosis. If must discontinue ADP receptor blocker, continue ASA and restart ADP receptor blocker ASAP.
- **β-blockers** (*Circ* 2009;120:2123; *JAMA* 2010;303:551; *Am J Med* 2012;125:953)
  - Continue βB in Pts on them chronically. Do not discontinue βB abruptly postop, as may cause sympathetic activation from withdrawal. Use IV agents peri-operatively if Pt unable to take PO.
  - In terms of initiating βB, conflicting evidence; may depend on how administered. Some studies show ↓ death & MI (*NEJM* 1996;335:1713 & 1999;341:1789), another showed ↑ MI, but ↑ death & stroke and ↑ bradycardia/HoTN (*Lancet* 2008;371:1839).
  - ? consider initiating if intermed- or high-risk ⊕ stress test, or RCRI ≥3, espec if vasc surgery
  - Ideally initiate at least 1 wk prior to surgery, use low-dose, short-acting βB, and titrate slowly and carefully to achieve desired individual HR and BP goal (? HR ~55–65). Avoid bradycardia and HoTN.
- **Statins:** ↓ ischemia & CV events in Pts undergoing vascular surg (*NEJM* 2009;361:980); may reduce AF, MI, LOS in statin-naïve Pts (*Arch Surg* 2012;147:181). Consider in Pts w/ a clinical risk factor undergoing non–low-risk surgery.
- **ACEI/ARB:** may cause HoTN perioperatively. If held before surgery, restart ASAP.
- **Amiodarone:** ↓ incidence of postop AF
  - oral (eg, 600 mg qd × 7 d preop, then 200 mg qd until discharge) & IV regimens equivalent but effective only if initiated ≥1 d prior to surgery (*Pacing Clin Electrophysiol* 2013;36:1017)
  - cardiac surgery: ↓ postop AF, length of stay & cost (*NEJM* 1997;337:1785)
  - thoracic surgery: ↓ postop AF but *not* length of stay or cost (*J Thorac CV Surg* 2010;140:45; *Ann Thorac Surg* 2012;94:339; *Eur J Cardiothorac Surg* 2014;45:120). Not advised if severe lung disease or undergoing pneumonectomy (*Ann Thorac Surg* 2011;92:1144).

Postoperative monitoring
- ✓ Postop ECG if known CAD or high-risk surgery. Consider if >1 risk factor for CAD.
- ✓ Postop troponin only if new ECG Δs or chest pain suggestive of ACS. Elevated Tn postop predicts mortality, but may simply be a marker for underlying CAD (*Annals* 2011;154:523; *JAMA* 2012;307:2295). Routine ✓ postop in all Pts (even just high-risk Pts) has not been proven to modify outcomes and it is not routinely recommended.

HEART FAILURE

Definitions (Braunwald's Heart Disease, 10th ed., 2014)
- Failure of heart to pump blood forward at sufficient rate to meet metabolic demands of peripheral tissues, or ability to do so only at abnormally high cardiac filling pressures
- Low output (↓ cardiac output) vs high output (↑ stroke volume ± ↑ cardiac output)
- Left-sided (pulmonary edema) vs right-sided (↑ JVP, hepatomegaly, peripheral edema)
- Backward (↑ filling pressures, congestion) vs forward (impaired systemic perfusion)
- Systolic (inability to expel sufficient blood) vs diastolic (failure to relax and fill normally)
- Reduced (HFrEF) vs preserved (HFpEF) left ventricular ejection fraction
- Some degree of systolic and diastolic dysfxn may occur regardless of ejection fraction

Figure 1-3 Approach to left-sided heart failure

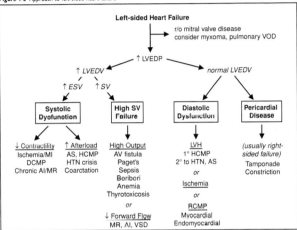

History
- Low output: fatigue, weakness, exercise intolerance, Δ MS, anorexia
- Congestive: dyspnea, weight gain;
  left-sided → orthopnea, paroxysmal nocturnal dyspnea
  right-sided → peripheral edema, RUQ discomfort, bloating, early satiety

Stages in the Development of Heart Failure (Circ 2009;119:e391)
- **A**: At high **risk for HF**, but w/o structural heart disease or symptoms of HF
- **B**: **Structural heart disease**, but w/o signs or symptoms of HF
- **C**: Structural heart disease w/ prior or current **symptoms of HF**
- **D**: **Refractory heart failure** requiring specialized intervention

Functional classification (New York Heart Association class)
- Class I: no sx w/ ordinary activity; class II: sx w/ ordinary activity;
  class III: sx w/ minimal activity; class IV: sx at rest

Physical exam ("2-minute" hemodynamic profile; JAMA 1996;275:630 & 2002;287:628)
- **Congestion ("dry" vs "wet")**:
  ↑ JVP (~80% of the time RAP >10 mmHg → PCWP >22 mmHg; JHLT 1999;18:1126)
  ⊕ hepatojugular reflux: ≥4 cm ↑ in JVP that persists for ≥15 sec w/ abdominal pressure
  Se/Sp 73/87% for RA >8 and Se/Sp 55/83% for PCWP >15 (AJC 1990;66:1002)
  Abnl Valsalva response: square wave (↑ SBP w/ strain), no overshoot (no ↑ BP after strain)
  S₃ (in Pts w/ HF → ~40% ↑ risk of HF hosp. or pump failure death; NEJM 2001;345:574)
  rales, dullness at base 2° pleural effus. (often absent in chronic HF due to lymphatic compensation) ± hepatomegaly, ascites and jaundice, peripheral edema
- **Perfusion ("warm" vs "cold")**: narrow pulse pressure (<25% of SBP) → CI <2.2 (91% Se, 83% Sp; JAMA 1989;261:884); other signs of low perfusion include soft S₁ (↓ dP/dt), pulsus alternans, cool & pale extremities, ↓ UOP, muscle atrophy
- Other signs to look for: periodic breathing/Cheyne-Stokes resp., abnl PMI (diffuse, sustained or lifting depending on cause of HF), S₄ (diast. dysfxn), murmur (valvular disease, ↑ MV or TV annulus, displaced papillary muscles), ↓ carotid upstroke

Evaluation for the presence of heart failure
- **CXR** (see Radiology insert): pulm edema, pleural effusions ± cardiomegaly, cephalization, Kerley B-lines
- **BNP/NT-proBNP** can help exclude HF; levels ↑ w/ age, renal dysfxn, AF, ↓ w/ obesity
  Se ≥95%, Sp ~50%, PPV ~65%, NPV ≥94% for HF in Pts p/w SOB (*BMJ* 2015;350:h910)
- Evidence of **↓ organ perfusion**: ↑ Cr, ↓ Na, abnl LFTs
- **Echo** (see inserts): ↓ EF & ↑ chamber size → systolic dysfxn; hypertrophy, abnl MV inflow, abnl tissue Doppler → ? diastolic dysfxn; abnl valves or pericardium; ↑ estimated RVSP
- **PA catheterization**: ↑ PCWP, ↓ CO & ↑ SVR (in low-output failure)

Evaluation of the potential causes of heart failure
- **ECG**: Q waves or PRWP (ischemic heart disease); LVH (hypertensive heart disease or HCM); low limb voltage (NICM or infiltrative); heart block (infiltrative)
- **TTE**: LV & RV size & function, valvular disease (and whether likely 1° or 2° to CMP); findings indicative of infiltrative or pericardial disease
- **Coronary angio** (or noninvasive imaging, eg, CT angio); if no CAD, w/u for NICM
- **Cardiac MRI**: multiparameter evaluation of cardiac structure & function including: LVEF, RVEF and volumes; regional wall motion abnormalities
  presence, pattern, & extent of myocardial scar (using late gadolinium enhancement, LGE) w/ Se/Sp of 100%/96% vs coronary angio for dx etiology of HF (*Circ* 2011;124:1351)
  myocardial inflammation or infiltration (eg, myocarditis, sarcoidosis, amyloidosis)
  restriction vs constrictive pericardial disease

Evaluation of Potential Causes of Heart Failure		
Etiology	**ECG Pattern**	**Imaging Pattern**
Ischemia, infarct	ST segment deviation, Qw	TTE: regional WMA, ± thinning/aneurysm Cor angio/CTA: obstructive CAD MRI: subendocardial or transmural LGE
Infiltrative	Low limb lead voltage, ± heart block, pseudoinfarct	TTE: LVH, "starry sky," ↑ biatrial size → amyloid MRI: inapprop nulling of myocardium + diffuse LGE → amyloid; patchy LV + RV LGE → sarcoidosis; ↓ T2 star → iron overload
Idiopathic DCM	Low limb lead volts, precordial LVH, BBB	TTE: 4 chamber dilation, diffuse hypokinesis MRI: mid-myocardial LGE
Tachy-myopathy	Persistent SVT	TTE: diffuse hypokinesis MRI: absent LGE in early stage
Myo(peri)-carditis	Pseudoischemia/-infarct. Pericard: diffuse concave STE w/ ST:T ratio >0.24 in V_6 and PR depression	TTE: typically global HK MRI: mid-myocardial + epicardial LGE, ↑ T2 and ↑ T1 ratios (edema)

Precipitants of acute heart failure
- **Dietary indiscretion or medical nonadherence** (~40% of cases)
- **Myocardial ischemia or infarction** (~10–15% of cases); myocarditis
- **Renal failure** (acute, progression of CKD, or insufficient dialysis) → ↑ preload
- **Hypertensive crisis** (incl. from RAS), **worsening AS** → ↑ left-sided afterload
- **Drugs** (βB, CCB, NSAIDs, TZDs), **chemo** (anthracyclines, trastuzumab), or **toxins** (EtOH)
- **Arrhythmias**; acute valv. dysfxn (eg, endocarditis), espec mitral or aortic regurgitation
- **COPD or PE** → ↑ right-sided afterload; **RV pacing**
- **Other**: extreme emotional stress; anemia, systemic infection, thyroid disease

Treatment of acute decompensated heart failure
- Assess degree of congestion & adequacy of perfusion
- For **congestion**: "LMNOP"
  Lasix IV w/ monitoring of UOP; total daily dose 2.5× usual daily PO dose → ↑ UOP, but transient ↑ in renal dysfxn vs 1× usual dose; ∅ clear diff between cont gtt vs q12h dosing (*NEJM* 2011;364:797)
  Morphine (↓ sx, venodilator, ↓ afterload)
  Nitrates (venodilator)
  Oxygen ± noninvasive vent (↓ sx, ↑ P_aO_2; no Δ mortality; see "Mechanical Ventilation")
  Position (sitting up & legs dangling over side of bed → ↓ preload)
- For **low perfusion**, see below

	Congestion?	
	No	**Yes**
No low perfusion	**Warm & Dry** *Outpatient Rx*	**Warm & Wet** *Diuresis*
Yes low perfusion	**Cold & Dry** *Inotropes (CCU)*	**Cold & Wet** *Diuresis, inotropes and/or vasodil (CCU)*

- Adjustment of oral meds
  ACEI/ARB: hold if HoTN, consider Δ to hydralazine & nitrates if renal decompensation
  βB: reduce dose by at least ½ if mod HF, d/c if severe HF and/or need inotropes

Overview of Treatment of Heart Failure by Stage		
Pt characteristics		**Therapy**
A	HTN, DM, CAD Cardiotoxin exposure FHx of CMP	Treat HTN, lipids, DM, SVT Stop smoking, EtOH; ↑ exercise ACEI/ARB if HTN/DM/CAD/PAD
B	Prior MI, ↓ EF, LVH or asx valvular dis.	All measures for stage A + ACEI/ ARB & βB if MI/CAD or ↓ EF. ? ICD.
C	Overt HF	All measures for stage A, ACEI, βB, diuretics, Na restrict ↓ EF: aldo antag, ICD, consider CRT, nitrate/hydral, dig.
D	Sx despite max med Rx 4-y mortality >50%	All measures for stages A–C Consider IV inotropes, VAD, transplant, end-of-life care

- Utility of BNP-guided Rx remains debated (Circ 2013;301:500 & 509)
- Implantable PA pressure sensor in NYHA III → 37% ↓ risk of hosp (23% for HFrEF; 52% for HFpEF) (Lancet 2011;377:658)

Treatment of advanced heart failure (Circ 2009;119:e391)
- Consider PAC (qv) if not resp to Rx, unsure re: vol status, HoTN, ↑ Cr, need inotropes
- Tailored Rx w/ PAC: goals of MAP >60, CI >2.2 (MVO₂ >60%), SVR <800, PCWP <18
- **IV vasodilators:** NTG, nitroprusside (risk of coronary steal if CAD; prolonged use → cyanide/thiocyanate toxicity); nesiritide (rBNP) not rec for routine use (NEJM 2011;365:32)
- **Inotropes:** in addition to ↑ inotropy, consider additional properties:
  dobutamine: vasodilation at doses ≤5 mcg/kg/min; mild ↓ PVR; desensitization over time
  dopamine: splanchnic vasodil. → ↑ GFR & natriuresis; vasoconstrictor at ≥5 mcg/kg/min;
  does not enhance decongestion or preserve renal fxn in ADHF (JAMA 2013;310:2533)
  milrinone: prominent systemic & pulmonary vasodilation; ↓ dose by 50% in renal failure
- Ultrafiltration: similar wt loss to aggressive diuresis, but ↑ renal failure (NEJM 2012;367:2296)
- **Mechanical circulatory support (MCS)** (JHLT 2013;32:157; JACC 2015;65:e7 & 2542)
  Temporary MCS: depending on the device (Table), can be placed percutaneously or surgically to support LV or RV as a bridge to recovery, for periprocedural support, or as a bridge to decision regarding transplant or durable long-term MCS
  Intra-aortic balloon pump (IABP): inflates in diastole & deflates in systole to ↓ impedance to LV ejection of blood, ↓ myocardial O₂ demand & ↑ coronary perfusion
  Axial flow pumps (eg, Impella): Archimedes screw principle in LV
  Extracorporeal magnetically levitated centrifugal pumps (eg, TandemHeart & CentraMag)
  Extracorporeal membrane oxygenation (ECMO, Circ 2015;131:676)

Short-Term Mechanical Circulatory Support in Cardiogenic Shock						
Device	**IABP**	**Impella 2.5 & CP**	**Impella 5.0**	**Tandem**	**CentriMag**	**ECMO**
Max support (L/min)	0.5	2.5 & 3–4	5.0	5.0	10	6
RV support	N	Y (2nd dev.)	N	Y (2nd dev.)	Y (2nd dev.)	Y
Support duration	wks	~4 wk	~4 wk	<4 wk	mos	wks
Percutan?	Y	Y	N	Y	N	Y
Contraindic.	≥ mod AI, severe PAD	LV thrombus, mech AV, severe AS		coagulop severe PAD	coagulop	coagulop

(Circ 2011;123:533 & 126:1717; JACC 2015;65:e7)

  Durable Long-term MCS: surgically placed LVAD ± RVAD as bridge to recovery (NEJM 2006;355:1873) or transplant (HeartMate II or HeartWare LVAD or Total Artificial Heart if biventricular failure), or as destination Rx (HeartMate I: 52% ↓ 1-y mort. vs med Rx; NEJM 2001;345:1435, HeartMate II: 24% ↓ mort. vs HeartMate 1; NEJM 2009;361:2241)
- **Cardiac transplantation:** curative Rx but supply of organs limited (~2500/y in U.S.)
  10% mortality in 1st year, median survival ~10 y
  Contraindications: active malignancy or infection, irreversible PHT (TPG>15, PVR>5WU despite pulmonary vasodilator Rx), active substance abuse or lack of social supports
  Relative contraindications: age (eg, >70 y), other end organ dysfunction (liver, kidney, lung, unless dual organ transplantation is performed)

Treatment of Chronic Heart Failure with Reduced Ejection Fraction

Diet, exercise	Na <2 g/d, fluid restriction, exercise training in ambulatory Pts
ACEI	↓ mortality: 40% in NYHA IV, 16% in NYHA II/III, 20–30% in asx but ↓ EF (NEJM 1992;327:685 & Lancet 2000;355:1575) High-dose more effic. than low. Watch for ↑ Cr, ↑ K (ameliorate by low-K diet, diuretics, Kayexalate; patiromer, another K binder, under review; NEJM 2015;372:211), cough, angioedema.
ATII receptor blockers (ARBs)	*Consider as alternative if cannot tolerate ACEI (eg, b/c cough)* Noninferior to ACEI (Lancet 2000;355:1582 & 2003;362:772) As with ACEI, higher doses more efficacious (Lancet 2009;374:1840) Adding to ACEI → ↑ risk of ↑ K and ↑ Cr (BMJ 2013;346:f360)
ARNi (ARB + neprilysin inhib)	Neutral endopeptidase (NEP, aka neprilysin) degrades natriuretic peptides as well as bradykinin & angiotensins. LCZ696 = valsartan + sacubitril (NEPi): ↓ CV mort & HF hosp c/w ACEi; more HoTN and trend to more angioedema (PARADIGM-HF, NEJM 2014;371:993).
Hydralazine + nitrates	*Consider if cannot tolerate ACEI/ARB or in blacks w/ NYHA III/IV* 25% ↓ mort. (NEJM 1986;314:1547); infer. to ACEI (NEJM 1991;325:303) 43% ↓ mort. in blacks on standard Rx (A-HEFT, NEJM 2004;351:2049)
β-blocker (data for carvedilol, metoprolol, bisoprolol)	EF will transiently ↓, then ↑. Contraindic. in decompensated HF. 35% ↓ mort. & 40% ↓ rehosp. in NYHA II–IV (NEJM 2002;287:883) Carvedilol superior to low-dose metop in 1 trial (Lancet 2003;362:7), but meta-analysis suggests no diff between βB (BMJ 2013;346:f55).
Aldosterone antagonists	*Consider if adeq. renal fxn and w/o hyperkalemia; watch for ↑ K* 24–30% ↓ mort. in NYHA II–IV & EF ≤35% (NEJM 2011;364:11) 15% ↓ mort. in post-MI, EF ≤40% (EPHESUS, NEJM 2003;348:1309)
Cardiac resynch therapy (CRT, qv)	*Consider if EF ≤35%, LBBB and symptomatic HF* 36% ↓ mort. & ↑ EF in NYHA III–IV (CARE-HF, NEJM 2005;352:1539) 41% ↓ mort. in EF ≤30%, LBBB and NYHA I/II (NEJM 2014;370:1694)
ICD (see "Cardiac Rhythm Mgmt Devices")	Use for 1° prevention if EF ≤30–35% or 2° prevention; not if NYHA IV ↓ mort. in ischemic & non-isch CMP; no Δ mort. early post-MI (NEJM 2004;351:2481 & 2009;361:1427), ∴ wait ≥40 d
Diuretics	Loop + thiazide diuretics (sx relief; no mortality benefit)
Digoxin	23% ↓ HF hosp., no Δ mort (NEJM 1997;336:525); ? ↑ mort w/ ↑ levels (NEJM 2002;347:1403); optimal 0.5–0.8 ng/mL (JAMA 2003;289:871)
Ivabradine (I_f blocker w/o ⊖ ino)	*Consider if HR >70, NSR on max βB.* 18% ↓ CV mort w/ HF hosp (Lancet 2010;376:875)
Ω-3 fatty acids	9% ↓ mortality (included HF with normal LVEF) (Lancet 2008;372:1223)
IV iron supplementation	? if NYHA II/III, EF ≤40%, Fe-defic (ferritin <100 or ferritin 100–300 & TSAT ↓20%). ↓ Sx, ↑ 6MWD, independent of Hct (NEJM 2009;361:2436).
Anticoagulation	*If AF, VTE, LV thrombus, ± if large akinetic LV segments* In SR w/ EF <35%, ↓ isch stroke, but ↑ bleed (NEJM 2012;366:1859)
Heart rhythm	Catheter ablation of AF → ↑ in EF, ↓ sx (NEJM 2004;351:2373) No mortality benefit to AF rhythm vs rate cntl (NEJM 2008;358:2667) Pulm vein isolation ↓ sx c/w AVN ablation & CRT (NEJM 2008;359:1778)
Meds to avoid	NSAIDs, nondihydropyridine CCB, TZDs
Experimental	Serelaxin ↓ dyspnea & ? ↓ mortality (Lancet 2013;381:29)

(Circ 2009;119:e391; NEJM 2010;362:228; Lancet 2011;378:713 & 722)

Heart failure with preserved EF (HFpEF; "Diastolic HF") (Circ 2011;124:e540)

- Epidemiology: ~½ of Pts w/ HF have normal or only min. impaired systolic fxn (EF ≥40%); risk factors for HFpEF incl ↑ age, ♀, DM, AF. Mortality ≈ those w/ systolic dysfxn.
- Etiologies (impaired relaxation and/or ↑ passive stiffness): ischemia, prior MI, LVH, HCMP, infiltrative CMP, RCMP, aging, hypothyroidism
- Precipitants of pulmonary edema: *volume overload* (poor compliance of LV → sensitive to even modest ↑ in volume); *ischemia* (↓ relaxation); *tachycardia* (↓ filling time in diastole); *AF* (loss of atrial boost to LV filling); *HTN* (↑ afterload → ↓ systole volume)
- Dx w/ clinical s/s of HF w/ preserved systolic fxn. Dx supported by evidence of diast dysfxn:
  (1) echo: abnl MV inflow (E/A reversal and Δs in E wave deceleration time) & ↓ myocardial relax. (↑ isovol relax. time & ↓ early diastole tissue Doppler velocities)
  (2) exercise-induced ↑ PCWP (± ↓ response chronotropic & vasodilator reserve)
- Treatment: diuresis for vol overload, BP control, prevention of tachycardia and ischemia; no benefit to: ACEI/ARB (NEJM 2008;359:2456) or PDE5 inhib (JAMA 2013;309:1268) spironolactone ↓ CV death & HF hosp (at least in Americas) (NEJM 2014;370:1383); ARNi (Lancet 2012;380:1387) and serelaxin (Lancet 2013;381:29) under study

PA CATHETER AND TAILORED THERAPY

Rationale
- Cardiac output (CO) = SV × HR; LV SV depends on LV end-diastolic volume (LVEDV) ∴ manipulate LVEDV to optimize CO while minimizing pulmonary edema
- Balloon at tip of catheter inflated → floats into "wedge" position. Column of blood extends from tip of catheter, through pulmonary circulation, to a point just proximal to LA. Under conditions of no flow, PCWP ≈ LA pressure ≈ LVEDP, which is proportional to LVEDV.
- Situations in which these basic assumptions fail:
  - (1) Catheter tip not in West lung zone 3 (and ∴ PCWP = alveolar pressure ≠ LA pressure); clues include lack of *a* & *v* waves and if PA diastolic pressure < PCWP
  - (2) PCWP > LA pressure (eg, mediastinal fibrosis, pulmonary VOD, PV stenosis)
  - (3) Mean LA pressure > LVEDP (eg, MR, MS)
  - (4) Δ LVEDP-LVEDV relationship (ie, abnl compliance, ∴ "nl" LVEDV may not be optimal)

Indications *(Circ 2009;119:e391; NEJM 2013;369:e35)*
- **Diagnosis and evaluation**
  - Ddx of shock (cardiogenic vs distributive; espec if trial of IVF failed or is high risk) and of pulmonary edema (cardiogenic vs not; espec if trial of diuretic failed or is high risk)
  - Evaluation of CO, intracardiac shunt, pulmonary HTN, MR, tamponade, cardiorenal syndrome
  - Evaluation of unexplained dyspnea (PAC during provocation w/ exercise, vasodilator)
- **Therapeutics** *(Circ 2006;113:1020)*
  - Tailored therapy to optimize PCWP, SV, $S_{MV}O_2$, RAP, & PVR, in heart failure or shock
  - Guide to vasodilator therapy (eg, Inhaled NO) In pulm HTN, RV Infarction
  - Guide to perioperative management in some high-risk Pts, pretransplantation
  - Guide to candidacy for thoracic organ transplantation and mechanical circulatory support
- **Contraindications**
  - **Absolute:** right-sided endocarditis, thrombus/mass or mechanical valve; PE
  - **Relative:** coagulopathy (reverse), recent PPM or ICD (place under fluoroscopy), LBBB (~5% risk of RBBB → CHB, place under fluoro), bioprosthetic R-sided valve

Efficacy concerns *(NEJM 2006;354:2213; JAMA 2005;294:1664)*
- No benefit to routine PAC use in high-risk surgery, sepsis, ARDS
- No benefit in decompensated HF *(JAMA 2005;294:1625)*; untested in cardiogenic shock
- But: ~1/2 of CO & PCWP clinical estimates incorrect; CVP & PCWP not well correl; ∴ use PAC to (a) answer hemodynamic ? and then remove, or (b) manage cardiogenic shock

Pulmonary Artery Catheter Features		
Component	**cm from distal tip**	**Function**
Distal lumen	0	Sampling of blood for $S_{MV}O_2$
1.5-mL balloon	0.5	Inflation allows flow directed placement & determination of PCWP
Thermistor	4	Detection of temp Δ for CO calc
Proximal injectate port	26	Infusions & injection of saline for CO calc
Additional Optional Features		
Fiberoptic O_2 sat sensor	0	Allows continuous measurement of $S_{MV}O_2$
Thermal filament	~10–25	Allows continuous CO calc by thermodilution
Pacing port	~19	Allows placement of pacing wire in RV
Infusion port(s)	~30	Additional infusion port(s)

Placement
- Insertion site: **R internal jugular** or **L subclavian** veins for "anatomic" flotation into PA
- **Inflate** balloon (max 1.5 mL) when **advancing** and to **measure PCWP**
- Use resistance to inflation and pressure tracing to avoid overinflation & risk of PA rupture
- Should require 1–1.5 mL air in balloon to float into wedge (<1 mL → pull PAC back; no PCWP at 1.5 mL → advance)
- **Deflate** balloon when **withdrawing** and at all other times
- CXR should be obtained after placement to assess for catheter position and PTX
- If catheter cannot be successfully floated (typically if severe TR or RV dilatation) or if another relative contraindication exists, use fluoroscopic guidance

Complications
- **Central venous access:** pneumo/hemothorax (~1%), arterial puncture (if inadvertent cannulation w/ dilation → surgical/endovasc eval), air embolism, thoracic duct injury
- **Arrhythmias:** 1/2 PVCs, 20% NSVT, 3% VT (minimize time PAC tip in RV); RBBB (5%)

- **Inability to advance:** difficulty RA → RV seen w/ lg RA and/or severe TR; difficulty RV → PA seen w/ lg RV; deflate balloon, withdraw 10 cm, inflate balloon & readvance. *If repeated attempts unsuccessful at bedside, then perform under fluoro (to avoid PAC coiling & potentially knotting, which would require interventional cardiology to extract).*
- **PA rupture:** risk factors include prolonged balloon inflation, PHT, anticoag. Presents w/ hemoptysis and, if severe, hypoxemia & hypovolemic shock. Keep balloon inflated, intubate w/ dbl-lumen endotracheal tube, lateral decubitus position with affected side down, STAT interventional radiology and/or thoracic surgery consultation.
- **Air embolism:** presents w/ dyspnea, chest pain, ↑ R-sided pressures, HoTN. *Place in Trendelenburg, high-flow O₂.*
- **Other:** infxn (espec if PAC >3 d old); thrombus; pulm infarction; valve/chordae damage

Intracardiac pressures

- Zero the transducer and level it with the right atrium (phlebostatic axis)
- Transmural pressure (≈ preload) = measured intracardiac pressure − intrathoracic pressure
- Intrathoracic pressure (usually slightly ⊖) is transmitted to vessels and heart
- **Always measure intracardiac pressure at end-expiration,** when intrathoracic pressure is closest to 0 ("high point" in spont. breathing Pts; "low point" in Pts on ⊕ pressure vent.)
- If ↑ intrathoracic pressure (eg, PEEP), measured PCWP *overestimates* true transmural pressures. Can approx by subtracting ~½ PEEP (× ¾ to convert cm H₂O to mmHg).
- PCWP: LV preload best estimated at *a* wave; risk of pulmonary edema from avg PCWP

Cardiac output

- **Thermodilution:** saline injected in RA. Δ in temp over time measured at thermistor (in PA) is integrated and is ≈ 1/CO. Inaccurate if ↓ CO, severe TR or shunt.
- **Fick method:** O₂ consumpt (VO₂) (L/min) = CO (L/min) × Δ arteriovenous O₂ content
  ∴ $CO = \dot{V}O_2/C(a-v)O_2$
  VO₂ ideally measured (espec if ↑ metab demands), but freq estimated (125 mL/min/m²)
  C(a-v)O₂ = [10 × 1.36 mL O₂/g of Hb × Hb g/dL × (S₂O₂−S$_{MV}$O₂)]
  S$_{MV}$O₂ is key variable that Δs with acute interventions
  If S$_{MV}$O₂ >80%, consider if the PAC is "wedged" (ie, pulm vein sat), L→R shunt, impaired O₂ utilization (severe sepsis, cyanide, carbon monoxide), ↑↑ FiO₂

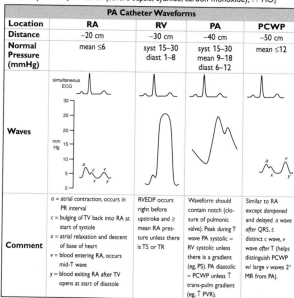

PA Catheter Waveforms				
Location	**RA**	**RV**	**PA**	**PCWP**
Distance	~20 cm	~30 cm	~40 cm	~50 cm
Normal Pressure (mmHg)	mean ≤6	syst 15–30 diast 1–8	syst 15–30 mean 9–18 diast 6–12	mean ≤12
Waves	simultaneous ECG			
Comment	*a* = atrial contraction, occurs in PR interval *c* = bulging of TV back into RA at start of systole *x* = atrial relaxation and descent of base of heart *v* = blood entering RA, occurs mid-T wave *y* = blood exiting RA after TV opens at start of diastole	RVEDP occurs right before upstroke and ≥ mean RA pressure unless there is TS or TR	Waveform should contain notch (closure of pulmonic valve). Peak during T wave PA systolic = RV systolic unless there is a gradient (eg, PS). PA diastolic ≈ PCWP unless ↑ trans-pulm gradient (eg, ↑ PVR).	Similar to RA except *dampened* and *delayed*. *a* wave *after* QRS, ± distinct *c* wave, *v* wave *after* T (helps distinguish MR from PA) w/ large *v* waves 2° MR from PA).

PCWP waveform abnormalities: large *a* wave → ? mitral stenosis; large *v* wave → ? mitral regurgitation; blunted *y* descent → ? tamponade; steep *x* & *y* descents → ? constriction.

Hemodynamic Profiles of Various Forms of Shock				
Type of shock	RA	PCWP	CO	SVR
Hypovolemic	↓	↓	↓	↑
Distributive	variable	variable	usually ↑ (but can be ↓ in sepsis)	↓
Cardiogenic: 1° L-sided (eg, acute MI)	nl or ↑	↑	↓	↑
Cardiogenic: 1° R-sided (eg, RV infarct; PE)	↑	nl or ↓	↓	↑
Tamponade	↑	↑	↓	↑

Surrogates: JVP ≈ RA; pulmonary edema on CXR implies ↑ PCWP; UOP ∝ CO (barring AKI); delayed capillary refill (ie, >2–3 sec) implies ↑ SVR

Tailored therapy and management of shock (Circ 2009;119:e391)
- **Goals:** optimize both MAP and CO to promote end-organ perfusion,
  while ↓ risk of pulmonary edema & systemic venous congestion
  MAP = CO × SVR; CO = HR × SV (depends on preload, afterload and contractility)
  pulmonary edema when PCWP >20–25 (↑ levels may be tolerated in chronic HF)
  hepatic and renal congestion when CVP/RAP >15 mmHg
- **Optimize preload** = LVEDV ≈ LVEDP ≈ LAP ≈ PCWP (NEJM 1973;289:1263)
  goal PCWP ~14–18 in acute MI, ≤14 in acute decompensated HF
  optimize in individual Pt by measuring SV w/ different PCWP to create Starling curve
  ↑ by giving NS (albumin w/o clinical benefit over NS; PRBC if significant anemia)
  ↓ by diuresis (qv), ultrafiltration or dialysis if refractory to diuretics
- **Optimize afterload** ≈ wall stress during LV ejection = [(~SBP × radius) / (2 × wall thick.)]
  and ∴ ∝ MAP and ∝ SVR = (MAP − CVP / CO); goals: **MAP >60, SVR 800–1200**
  MAP >60 & SVR ↑: vasodilators (eg, nitroprusside, NTG, ACEI, hydral.) or wean pressors
  MAP <60 & SVR ↑ (& ∴ CO ↓): temporize w/ pressors until can ↑ CO (see below)
  MAP <60 & SVR low/nl (& ∴ inappropriate vasoplegia): vasopressors (eg, norepineph-rine [α, β], dopamine [D, α, β], phenylephrine [α] or vasopressin [V₁] if refractory)
- **Optimize contractility** ∝ CO for given preload & afterload; **goal CI = (CO / BSA) >2.2**
  if too low despite optimal preload & vasodilators (as MAP permits):
    ⊕ inotropes: eg, dobutamine (mod inotrope & mild vasodilator) or milrinone (strong inotrope & vasodilator, incl pulm), both proarrhythmic, or epi (strong inotrope & pressor)
    mechanical support devices: eg, IABP, percutaneous or surgical VAD (L-sided, R-sided, or both) or ECMO (Circ 2011;123:533)

Vasopressors and Inotropes Used in Shock							
Drug	Receptors			Hemodynamics				Comment
	α₁	β₁	β₂	SVR	MAP	HR	CO	
Phenylephrine	+++	0	0	↑↑↑	↑↑	↓↓ᵃ	↓ᵃ	↑ PVR
Vasopressinᵇ	0	0	0	↑↑↑	↑↑	↓↓ᵃ	↓ᵃ	↔ PVR; ∴ attractive if RV dysfxn or PHT
Norepinephrine	+++	++	+	↑↑↑	↑↑	↔/↑	↔/↑	Better outcomes than w/ dopa
Epinephrine	+++	+++	+++	↓ / ↑ᶜ	↑	↑↑	↑	β predom at low doses
Isoproterenol	0	+++	+++	↓↓	↓	↑↑↑	↑↑	⊕ chronotrope
Dobutamine	+	+++	++	↓	↔/↓	↑↑	↑↑	↓ PCWP
Dopamineᵈ	+	++	0	↔/↑ᵈ	↔/↑ᵈ	↑↑↑	↑	
Milrinoneᵉ	0	0	0	↓↓	↓	↔	↑↑↑	↓↓ PCWP; ↓ PVR; ∴ attractive if RV dysfxn or PHT

ᵃBradycardia seen due to vagal reflex if hypertension; ↓ CO due to ↑ afterload
ᵇV₁ agonist
ᶜLow doses ↓ SVR, high doses ↑ SVR
ᵈAlso a (D) dopa receptor agonist; 0.5–2 mcg/kg/min → D; 2–10 → D & β₁; >10 → α₁, β₁, D
ᵉPDE₃ inhibitor

Diseases with mechanical and/or electrical dysfunction of the myocardium

DILATED CARDIOMYOPATHY (DCM)

Definition and epidemiology *(Circ 2013;128:e240; JACC 2013;62:2046)*
- Ventricular dilatation and ↓ contractility ± ↓ wall thickness *in the absence of myocardial disease* caused by ischemia/infarct, valvular disease or hypertension
- Ventricular dysfunction usually global but can be regional variation
- May be accompanied by significant MR & TR due to impaired leaflet coaptation
- Incidence: 5–8/100,000/y; prevalence: 1/2500. Most common reason for heart transplant.

Etiologies *(JACC 2011;57:1641; Circ Res 2012;111:131)*
- **Familial** (>35%): defined as having DCM and at least 2 closely related family members with otherwise unexplained DCM; usually autosomal dominant pattern of inheritance; ~30 genes identified to date, encoding structural & nuclear proteins
  sarcomere: eg, titin (*TTN*, ~20%; *NEJM* 2012;366:619); β- & α-myosin heavy chain (*MYH7, MYH6*, ~5% each); troponin T (*TNNT2*, ~5%)
  nuclear envelope: eg, lamin A/C (*LMNA*, ~5%), often w/ conduction system disease (eg, sinus brady, AV block, atrial arrhythmias) *(NEJM 2009;341:1715)*
  ion channel: eg, Na channel (*SCN5A*, <5%), same gene as for LQTS & Brugada
  Z-disc: eg, myopalladin (*MYPN*, <5%), ankyrin (*ANKRD1*, <5%)
  cytoskeletal: eg, desmin (*DES*, <1%); dystrophin (*DMD*, <1%)
  syndromic disorders: eg, muscular dystrophies (Duchenne/Becker; limb-girdle)
- **Idiopathic** (<20%): ? undiagnosed infectious, alcoholic or genetic cause (in ~1/4 of Pts w/ "idiopathic" DCM, evidence of DCM found in 1° relative, suggesting undx genetic)
- **Infectious myocarditis** (10–15%, autoimmune response; *Lancet 2012;379:738*)
  Viruses (parvoB19 & HHV6 > coxsackie, adeno, CMV, HCV): from subacute (dilated LV; mild–mod dysfxn) to fulminant (nondil., thick, edematous LV; sev dysfxn)
  Bacterial, fungal, rickettsial, TB, Lyme (mild myocarditis, often with AVB, qv)
  HIV: ~8% of asx HIV ⊕; due to HIV, 2° infxns, or antiretrovirals; HIV also associated w/ premature CAD *(JACC 2012;59:779)*
  Chagas: apical aneurysm ± thrombus, RBBB, megaesophagus/colon *(NEJM 2015;373:456)*
- **Toxic**
  alcohol (20–35%; *Prog CV Dis 2010;52:289*): typically 7–8 drinks/d × >5 y, but variable; male > female, typical age 30–55, may resolve w/ abstinence
  cocaine (primarily myocardial ischemia, but DCM is also seen); amphetamines & ephedra; anabolic steroids
  XRT (usually RCM); cobalt; chloroquine
  anthracyclines: risk ↑ >550 mg/m², may manifest late; usually irreversible
  cyclophosphamide, taxoids, mitomycin-C, 5-fluorouracil, and interferons
  trastuzumab: usually reversible
- **Infiltrative** (5%): often mix of DCM + RCM (qv) with thickened walls
  sarcoidosis, amyloidosis, hemochromatosis, tumor
- **Autoimmune**
  collagen vasc. dis./vasculitis (~5%): PM, SLE, scleroderma, PAN, RA, Wegener's;
  peripartum (last month → 5 mo postpartum; *EHJ 2015;36:1090*): ~1:3000 preg. ↑ risk w/ multiparity, ↑ age, Afr Am; stnd HF Rx except if preg then select drugs based on safety; ? bromocriptine to ↓ prolactin; 72% normalize EF; predictors of poor recovery include EF <30% & LVEDD ≥6 cm *(JACC 2015;66:905)*; even if nl EF, ~30% recur w/ next preg
  idiopathic giant cell myocarditis (GCM): avg age 42 y, may present as severe HF, high-grade AV block, or VT, historically poor prognosis (<6 mo median transplant-free survival; *NEJM 1997;336:1860*), but with modern immunosuppression 67% achieve HF remission with transplant-free survival of 77% at 1 y *(Circ HF 2013;6:15)*
  eosinophilic (variable peripheral eos): hypersensitivity (mild HF but at risk for SCD) or acute necrotizing eosinophilic myocarditis (ANEM; STE, effusion, severe HF)
- **Stress-induced** (Takotsubo = apical ballooning)
  typically seen in postmenopausal ♀ after psychological stressor
  ? due to catecholamine surge → microvasc dysfxn & Ca overload
  mimics MI (pain, ± STE & ↑ Tn; deep TWI & ↑ QT); mid/apex dyskinesis, sometimes w/ cardiogenic shock (caution w/ pressors as can induce LV outflow tract obstruction)
  ? Rx w/ βB, ACEI, anticoag if LV thrombus (but usually not just for dyskinesis given rapid resolution); usually improves over wks *(JAMA 2011;306:277)*
- **Tachycardia:** likelihood ∝ duration & rate (although avg HR ~120); often resolves w/ rate control, which is only way to definitely make dx, over several mos *(Circ 2005;112:1092)*
- **Arrhythmogenic (right ventricular) cardiomyopathy** (ACM, formerly ARVC): see below

- **Metabolic/other**
  hypothyroidism, acromegaly, pheo; OSA; cirrhosis
  thiamine, selenium or carnitine deficiency
- **LV noncompaction:** see below

Clinical manifestations
- **Heart failure:** both congestive & poor forward flow sx; signs of L- & R-sided HF
  diffuse, laterally displaced PMI, S3, ± MR or TR (annular dilat., displaced pap. muscle)
- Embolic events (~10%), supraventricular/ventricular arrhythmias, & palpitations
- Chest pain can be seen w/ some etiologies (eg, myocarditis)

Diagnostic studies and workup
- CXR: moderate to marked cardiomegaly, ± pulmonary edema & pleural effusions
- ECG: may see PRWP, Q waves or BBB; low-voltage; AF (20%); may be normal
- Echocardiogram: LV dilatation, ↓ EF, regional or global LV HK ± RV HK, ± mural thrombi
- Cardiac MRI: up to 76% Se, 96% Sp for myocarditis or infiltrative disease (*JACC Imaging* 2014;7:254); nontransmural delayed gadolinium enhancement in noncoronary distribution suggestive of DCM; extent of midwall fibrosis correlated w/ mortality in NICM (*JAMA* 2013;309:896)
- Laboratory evaluation: TFTs, iron studies, HIV, SPEP, ANA; others per clinical suspicion; viral serologies not recommended (*JACC* 2012;59:779)
- Stress test: useful to r/o ischemia (low false ⊖ rate), high false ⊕ rate, even w/ imaging
- Coronary angiography to r/o CAD if risk factors, h/o angina, Qw MI on ECG, equivocal ETT; consider CT angiography (*JACC* 2007;49:2044)
- ? Endomyocardial biopsy (*JACC* 2007;50:1914)
  yield 10% of these, 75% myocarditis (for which no proven Rx) & 25% systemic disease 40% false ⊖ rate (patchy dis.) & false ⊕ (necrosis → inflammation)
  ∴ biopsy if: acute & hemodynamic or electrical compromise (r/o GCM, ANEM); arrhythmia or RCMP features (r/o infiltrative); or suspect toxic, allergic, tumor
- Family hx & genetic testing (*JAMA* 2009;302:2471; *Circ* 2013;128:e240)
  family hx for ≥3 generations; incomplete penetrance and variable expression make dx of familial CMP challenging
  sequencing of DCM gene panels now available; typically test most clearly affected person
  if specific mutation identified, then can screen family using genetic testing
  if no mutation identified, consider cascade clinical screening (ECG, echo) of 1° relatives every ~3–5 years

Treatment (see "Heart Failure" for standard HF Rx)
- Implantation of devices may be tempered by possibility of reversibility of CMP
- Immunosuppression: for giant cell myocarditis (prednisone + AZA + cyclosporine), collagen vasc disease, peripartum (? IVIg), & eosinophilic; no proven benefit for viral myocarditis
- Prognosis differs by etiology (*NEJM* 2000;342:1077): postpartum (best), ischemic/GCM (worst)
- Abstain from EtOH (for alcoholic CMP and reasonable for others)
- Consider ACEI and/or βB if genotype ⊕ but currently phenotype ⊖

HYPERTROPHIC CARDIOMYOPATHY (HCM)

Definition and epidemiology
- LV (usually ≥15 mm) and/or RV hypertrophy disproportionate to hemodynamic load
- Prevalence: 1/500; 50% sporadic, 50% familial, most asymptomatic
- Autosomal-dominant mutations (>1500) in cardiac sarcomere genes
  most common genes involved: β-myosin heavy chain (*MYH7*, ~40%), myosin-binding protein C (*MYBPC3*, ~40%), cardiac troponin T (*TNNT2*, ~5%) and I (*TNNI3*, ~5%)
  no clear correlation between genotype and clinical course
- Noonan syndrome: HCM, pulmonic stenosis, ASD, short stature, pectus, webbed neck
- Ddx: LVH 2° to HTN, AS, elite athletes (wall usually <13 mm & symmetric and nl/↑ rates of tissue Doppler diastolic relaxation; LV cavity large; no late gadolinium enhancement on MRI; *Circ* 2011;123:2723), Fabry dis. (↑ Cr, skin findings)

Pathology
- Myocardial fiber disarray with hypertrophy, which creates arrhythmogenic substrate
- Morphologic hypertrophy variants: asymmetric septal; concentric; midcavity; apical
- LVH evolves over time, typically manifests in adolescence

Pathophysiology
- Subaortic outflow obstruction: narrowed tract 2° hypertrophied septum + systolic anterior motion (SAM) of ant. MV leaflet (may be fixed, variable or nonexistent) and papillary muscle displacement. Gradient (∇) worse w/ ↑ contractility (digoxin, β-agonists, exercise, PVCs), ↓ preload or ↓ afterload.

- Mitral regurgitation: due to SAM (mid-to-late, post.-directed regurg. jet) and/or abnl mitral leaflets and papillary muscles (pansystolic, ant.-directed regurg. jet)
- Diastolic dysfunction: ↑ chamber stiffness + impaired relaxation
- Ischemia: small vessel dis., perforating artery compression (bridging), ↓ coronary perfusion
- Syncope: Δs in load-dependent CO, arrhythmias

Clinical manifestations (70% asymptomatic at dx)
- **Dyspnea** (90%): due to ↑ LVEDP, MR, and diastolic dysfunction
- **Angina** (25%) even w/o epicardial CAD; microvasc. dysfxn (NEJM 2003;349:1027)
- **Arrhythmias** (AF in 20–25%;VT/VF) → palpitations, syncope, sudden cardiac death

Physical exam
- Sustained PMI, S_2 paradoxically split if severe outflow obstruction, ⊕ S_4 (occ. palpable)
- **Systolic murmur:** crescendo-decrescendo; LLSB; ↑ **w/ Valsalva** & standing (↓ preload)
- ± mid-to-late or holosystolic murmur of MR at apex
- Bifid carotid pulse (brisk rise, decline, then 2nd rise); JVP w/ prominent a wave
- Contrast to AS, which has murmur that ↓ w/ Valsalva and ↓ carotid pulses

Diagnostic studies
- CXR: cardiomegaly (LV and LA)
- ECG: LVH, anterolateral and inferior pseudo-Qw, ± apical giant TWI (apical variant)
- Echo: no absolute cutoffs for degree of LVH but septum/post. wall ≥1.3 suggestive, as is septum >15 mm; other findings include dynamic outflow obstruction, SAM, MR
- MRI: hypertrophy + patchy delayed enhancement (useful for dx & prog) (Circ 2015;132:292)
- Cardiac cath: subaortic pressure ∇; Brockenbrough sign = ↓ pulse pressure post-PVC (in contrast to AS, in which pulse pressure ↑ post-PVC)
- ? Genotyping for family screening, but pathogenic mutation ID'd in <¹/₂ (Circ 2011;124:2761)

Treatment (Circ 2011;124:e783 & 2012;125:1432; Lancet 2013;381:242; EHJ 2014;35:2733)
- Heart failure
  ⊖ **inotropes/chronotropes:** nonvasodilating βBs, CCB (verapamil), disopyramide Careful use of diuretics, as may further ↓ preload.Vasodilators only if systolic dysfxn. Avoid digoxin.
  If sx refractory to drug Rx + obstructive physiology (∇ >50 mmHg):
  (a) Surgical myectomy: long-term ↑ symptoms in 90% (Circ 2014;130:1617)
  (b) Alcohol septal ablation (Circ CV Interv 2011;4:256; JACC 2011;58:2322): gradient ↓ by ~80%, only 5–20% remain w/ NYHA III–IV sx; 14% require repeat ablation or myectomy. Good alternative for older Pts, multiple comorbidities. Complic: transient (& occ. delayed) 3° AVB w/ 10–20% req. PPM;VT due to scar formation.
  No clear benefit of dual-chamber pacing (JACC 1997;29:435; Circ 1999;99:2927)
  If refractory to drug therapy and there is nonobstructive pathophysiology: transplant
- Acute HF: can be precip. by dehydration or tachycardia; Rx w/ fluids, βB, phenylephrine
- AF: rate control with βB, maintain SR with disopyramide, amiodarone; low threshold to anticoagulate
- SCD: ICD (JACC 2003;42:1687). Risk factors: h/o VT/VF, ⊕ FHx SCD, unexplained syncope, NSVT, ↓ SBP or rel HoTN (↑ SBP <20 mmHg) w/ exercise, LV wall ≥30 mm, extensive MRI delayed enhancement. EPS not useful. Risk 11%/y if h/o VT/VF, 4%/y if high-risk w/o h/o VT/VF (JAMA 2007;298:405).
- Counsel to avoid dehydration, competitive sports & extreme exertion
- Endocarditis prophylaxis not recommended (Circ 2007;116:1736)
- First-degree relatives: periodic screening w/ echo, ECG (as timing of HCM onset variable). Genetic testing if known mutation. ? CCB for preclinical HCM (JACC HF 2015;3:180).

RESTRICTIVE CARDIOMYOPATHIES (RCM)

Definition (Circ 2006;113:1807)
- Impaired ventricular filling with ↓ compliance in nonhypertrophied, nondilated ventricles; normal or ↓ diastolic volumes, normal or near-normal EF; must r/o pericardial disease

Amyloidosis (Circ 2011;124:1079 & 2012:126:1286)
- Extracellular deposition of misfolded proteins in a variety of organs (eg, heart, kidney, liver, autonomic nervous system; deposition leads to morbidity & mortality)
- Age at presentation ~60 y; ♂:♀ = 3:2
- AL (primary; MM, light-chain, MGUS,WM): multiorgan disease (~50% cardiac)
- ATTR (familial; mutation in transthyretin, TTR; Circ 2012;126:1286)
  V122I variant ~2.6× ↑ HF risk; 10% carriage in blacks >65 y w/ HF (JACC 2006;47:1724)
  V30M variant seen in European & Japanese
  T60R variant in Europeans, autonomic + peripheral neuropathy common

- SSA (senile; normal TTR): typically presents at age >70 y, prevalence >5% beyond age 80, ♂ >> ♀ (50:1), heart-only
- Workup
  - ECG: ↓ QRS amplitude in AL (50%), pseudoinfarct pattern (Qw), AVB (10–20%), hemiblock (20%), BBB (5–20%)
  - Echo: biventricular wall thickening (yet w/ low voltage on ECG), granular sparkling texture (30%), biatrial enlargement (40%), thickened atrial septum, valve thickening (65%), diastolic dysfxn, small effusions
    Normal voltage & septal thickness has NPV ~90%
  - Lab: SPEP, UPEP, serum free light chain ratio (<0.25 or >1.65 κ-to-λ ratio) 91% Se for AL amyloid (Clin Chem 2005;51:878)
  - MRI: diffuse subendo late gado enhance, ~90% Se/Sp vs bx (JACC 2008;51:1022)
  - (99m)Tc-pyrophosphate PET: ↑ tracer retention in ATTR >> AL differentiates cardiac amyloid subtypes (Circ Imaging 2013;6:195)
  - Cardiac bx: gold standard (~100% Se due to widespread amyloid distrib) and permits subtyping of precursor protein. Abd fat pad bx 70% sensitivity for AL.
- Treatment: judicious loop diuretics often only tolerated Rx
  avoid digoxin (↑ toxicity w/ binding fibrils) and CCB (⊖ inotrope)
  βB or ACEI often poorly tolerated b/c of HoTN
  cardiac tx usually contraindic. b/c extracardiac involvement, but isolated cardiac AL amyloid combined heart/auto stem cell tx yields survival ≈ other RCM (JHLT 2014;33:149)
  LVADs not appropriate b/c small restricted LV and frequent RV dysfunction
- Prognosis (median survival after HF dx): AL <12 mo, ATTR ~30 mo, SSA ~60 mo

Sarcoidosis
- Noncaseating, granulomatous disorder that can involve any organ
- Recognized cardiac disease in ~5% of those w/ systemic sarcoid, but imaging & autopsy data show myocardial involvement in >50%
- LV dysfxn (DCM ≥ RCM); MR can be due to involvement of papillary muscles
- ECG: AVB (75%), can be high grade; RBBB (20–60%); atrial & vent. arrhythmias
- Cardiac MRI: T2-imaging and early gadolinium detect acute inflammation (edema), nontransmural patchy delayed gado enhancement, particularly in basal and/or midventricular septum detects fibrosis/scar from chronic disease and predicts prognosis (⊕ LGE → 31× risk for adverse cardiac events, JACC Imaging 2013;6:501)
- Echo: regional WMA (particularly basal septum) with thinning or mild hypertrophy
- Nuclear imaging: thallium perfusion defects in a noncoronary distribution, gallium uptake in areas of active inflammation can guide steroid Rx; PET: ↑ FDG uptake in areas of active inflammation
- Cardiac bx w/ low yield as granulomas patchy
- Treatment: steroids are standard although have not been evaluated in RCTs; 47% of Pts w/ AV conduction disease improved w/ steroids (Can J Cardiol 2013;29:1034) and retrospective studies suggest ↓ mortality. For steroid-sparing or intolerance, consider MTX, AZA, chloroquine or anti-TNF drugs. Low threshold for PPM-ICD.

Hemochromatosis
- In middle-aged men (espec Northern European)
- 15% p/w cardiac sx, typically HF and conduction disturbances
- Cardiac MRI: myocardial T2* is reduced (<20 ms) in iron overload disorders and enables tracking of response to Rx
- Treatment w/ phlebotomy or, in one report, chelation has been associated with reversal of LV dysfunction (JACC 1986;8:436)

Other etiologies (Circ 2005;112:2047 & JACC 2010;55:1769)
- **Myocardial processes**
  Autoimmune (scleroderma, polymyositis-dermatomyositis)
  Infiltrative diseases (see primary entries for extracardiac manifestations, Dx, Rx)
  Storage diseases: Gaucher's, Fabry, Hurler's, glycogen storage diseases
  Diabetes mellitus
- **Endomyocardial processes**
  Chronic eosinophilic: Löffler's endocarditis (temperate climates; ↑ eos; mural thrombi that embolize); endomyocardial fibrosis (tropical climates; var. eos; mural thrombi; NEJM 2008;359:43); treat for heart failure, steroids early, anticoagulation for thrombus
  Toxins: radiation (also p/w constrictive pericarditis, valvular dis, ostial CAD), anthracyclines
  Serotonin: carcinoid, serotonin agonists, ergot alkaloids
  Metastatic cancer

Pathology & pathophysiology
- Path: normal or ↑ wall thickness ± infiltration or abnormal deposition
- ↓ myocardial compliance → nl EDV but ↑ EDP → ↑ systemic & pulm. venous pressures
- ↓ ventricular cavity size → ↓ SV and ↓ CO

Clinical manifestations (Circ 2000;101:2490)
- **Right-sided > left-sided heart failure** w/ peripheral edema ± ascites > pulmonary edema
- Diuretic **"refractoriness"**
- **Thromboembolic events**
- Poorly tolerated tachyarrhythmias; VT → syncope/sudden cardiac death

Physical exam
- ↑ JVP, ± Kussmaul's sign (JVP ↑ w/ inspiration, classically seen in *constrictive pericarditis*)
- Cardiac: ± S₃ and S₄ (usually absent in amyloid b/c atrial dysfxn), ± murmurs of MR and TR
- Congestive hepatomegaly, ± ascites and jaundice, peripheral edema

Diagnostic studies
- CXR: normal ventricular chamber size, enlarged atria, ± pulmonary congestion
- ECG: low voltage, pseudoinfarction pattern (Qw), ± arrhythmias
- Echo: ± symmetric wall thickening, biatrial enlarge., ± mural thrombi, ± cavity oblit. w/ diast dysfxn: ↑ early diast (E) and ↓ late atrial (A) filling, ↑ E/A ratio, ↓ decel. time
- Cardiac MRI/PET: may reveal inflammation or evidence of infiltration (but nonspecific)
- Initials labs: SPEP, UPEP & serum free light chains. Fe studies (transferrin sat, HFE mutation), BNP (typically higher in RCM than in constrictive pericarditis)
- Cardiac catheterization: atria: **M's** or **W's** (prominent x and y descents)
  Ventricles: **dip & plateau** (rapid ↓ pressure at onset of diastole, rapid ↑ to early plateau)
  Concordance of LV and RV pressure peaks during respiratory cycle (vs discordance in constrictive pericarditis; Circ 1996;93:2007)
- Endomyocardial biopsy if suspect infiltrative process; fat pad bx for amyloid
- Restrictive cardiomyopathy vs constrictive pericarditis: see "Pericardial Disease"

Treatment (in addition to Rx'ing underlying disease)
- Gentle diuresis. May not tolerate CCB or other vasodilators. Avoid digoxin in amyloid.
- Control HR (but can ↓ CO); maintain SR (helps filling). Digoxin ↑ arrhythmias in amyloid.
- Inotropes may have limited efficacy due to small ventricular cavity & preserved systolic fxn
- Anticoagulation (particularly with AF or low CO)
- Transplantation for refractory cases

OTHER CARDIOMYOPATHIES

Arrhythmogenic (right ventricular) cardiomyopathy (ACM, formerly ARVC)
- RV or biventricular (~50%) or isolated LV (rare) dysfxn due to fatty infiltration and fibrous replacement (small amount of former normal variant) (Lancet 2009;373:1289)
- Due to mutations in desmosome (cell-cell coupling): eg, plakophilin 2, desmoglein, desmo-plakin; abnl Wnt signaling leads to myocytes → adipocytes
- Naxos syndrome (mutation in plakoglobin): wooly hair, palmar & plantar keratoses, ACM
- Clinical phases (Circ CV Gen 2015;8:437): (1) subclinical w/ nl imaging, but ↑ risk of SCD; (2) abnl ventricular fxn on imaging, sx ventricular arrhythmias (VT w/ LBBB morphology w/ superior axis), but no HF; (3) RV failure; (4) ? LV failure
- ECG: ± RBBB, TWI V₁–V₃, ε wave V₂ Epsilon
- Dx w/ MRI

- Avoid bx as septum usually *not* involved (∴ high false ⊖ rate) and risk of perforation w/ free wall bx
- Major dx criteria (EHJ 2010;31:806): (1) regional RV akinesia/dyskinesia and ↑ RVEDV; (2) fibrous replacement of RV free wall; (3) TWI V₁–V₃, (4) ε wave
- Treatment (Circ 2015;132:441): usual HF Rx; EP study & ICD; VT ablation as needed

Ion channelopathies (CMP despite lack of structural abnl; Circ 2006;113:1807)
- Defective ionic channel proteins lead to abnl cell membrane transit of Na and K ions
- Disorders include: LQTS, short-QT syndrome (SQTS), Brugada syndrome, and catecholaminergic polymorphic ventricular tachycardia (CPVT)

LV noncompaction (LVNC; JACC 2015;66:578)
- Prominent trabeculae w/ deep intertrabecular recesses due to intrauterine arrest of compaction of loose interwoven myocardial meshwork
- Debated whether distinct genetic abnl vs morphological trait of other CMPs
- Clinical: HF, atrial and/or vent arrhythmias, cardioembolic events
- Dx w/ MRI > echo; >2:1 ratio of noncompacted to compacted myocardium at end-systole, thickened LV wall and prominent deep trabeculae
- Usual HF Rx; low threshold to anticoagulate

AORTIC STENOSIS (AS)

Etiology
- **Calcific:** predominant cause in Pts >70 y; risk factors include HTN, ↑ chol., ESRD
- **Congenital** (ie, bicuspid AoV w/ premature calcification): cause in 50% of Pts <70 y
- **Rheumatic heart disease** (AS usually accompanied by AR and MV disease)
- AS mimickers: subvalvular (HCMP, subAo membrane) or supravalvular stenosis

Clinical manifestations (usually indicates AVA <1 cm² or concomitant CAD)
- **Angina:** ↑ O_2 demand (hypertrophy) + ↓ O_2 supply (↓ cor perfusion pressure) ± CAD
- **Syncope** (*exertional*): peripheral vasodil. w/ fixed CO → ↓ MAP → ↓ cerebral perfusion
- **Heart failure:** outflow obstruct + diastolic dysfxn → pulm. edema; espec If ↑ HR/AF (↓ LV fill.)
- Acquired vWF disease (~20% of sev. AS): destruction of vWF; GI angiodysplasia
- Natural hx: usually slowly progressive (AVA ↓ ~0.1 cm²/y, but varies; *Circ* 1997;95:2262), until sx develop; mean survival based on sx: angina = 5 y; syncope = 3 y; CHF = 2 y

Physical exam
- **Midsystolic crescendo-decrescendo** murmur at **RUSB,** harsh, high-pitched, radiates to carotids, apex (holosystolic = Gallavardin effect), ↑ w/ passive leg raise, ↓ w/ standing & Valsalva. In contrast, dynamic outflow obstruction (HCM) ↓ w/ leg raise, ↑ w/ standing, Valsalva.
- Ejection click after S_1 sometimes heard with *bicuspid* AoV
- Signs of severity: *late-peaking* murmur, paradoxically split S_2 or inaudible A_2, small and delayed carotid pulse ("*pulsus parvus et tardus*"), LV heave, ⊕ S_4 (occasionally palpable)

Diagnostic studies
- **ECG:** may see LVH, LAE, LBBB, AF (in late disease)
- **CXR:** cardiomegaly, AoV calcification, poststenotic dilation of ascending Ao, pulmonary congestion
- **Echo:** valve morphology, jet velocity, estim pressure gradient (∇) & calculate AVA, LVEF if concom severe AR: vel & ∇ may be ↑ than typical b/c of ↑ flow, but AVA calc valid if concom severe MR: vel & ∇ may be ↓ than typical b/c of ↓ flow, but AVA calc valid
- **Cardiac cath:** usually to r/o CAD (in ~¹/₂ of calcific AS), for hemodyn. if disparity between exam & echo: ✓ pressure gradient (∇) across AoV, calc AVA (underestim. if mod/sev AR)
- **Dobutamine challenge:** in cases with low flow, low ∇, and low LVEF, repeating echo (or cath) during low-dose dobutamine can differentiate:

Pathophys Heart Dis., 5th ed., 2010, for this et al.

Condition	Comment	SV	Jet Vel	∇	AVA
Afterload mismatch	Low EF 2° to severe AS; EF should ↑ post-AVR	≥20% ↑	↑	↑	no Δ
Pseudostenosis	Low AVA *artifact* of LV dysfxn	≥20% ↑	no Δ	no Δ	↑
Lack contractile reserve	EF prob. will *not* ↑ w/ AVR	no Δ	no Δ	no Δ	no Δ

Classification of Aortic Stenosis (*Circ* 2014;129:e521)						
Stage	Sx	Severity	Max Jet Vel (ᵐ/ₛ)	Mean Grad (mmHg)	AVA (cm²)ᵃ	LVEF
n/a	N	Normal	1	0	3–4	nl
A	N	At risk	<2	<10	3–4	nl
B	N	Mild	2–2.9	<20	>1.5	nl
		Moderate	3–3.9	20–39	1–1.5	nl
C1	N	Severe	≥4	≥40	≤1.0	nl
		Very severe	≥5	≥60	≤0.8	nl
C2		Severe + ↓ EF	≥4	≥40	≤1.0	↓
D1		Severe	≥4	≥40	≤1.0	nl
D2	Y	Severe + low flow/∇ + ↓ EFᵇ	<4	<40	≤1.0	↓
D3		Severe + low flow/∇ + nl EFᶜ	<4	<40	≤1.0	nl

ᵃAVA indexed to BSA <0.6 cm²/m² also severe; ᵇDSE → max jet vel ≥4 & AVA ≤1.0; ᶜsmall LV w/ ↓ stroke vol.

Treatment (*Circ* 2014;129:e521 & *NEJM* 2014;371:744)

- Management decisions based on *symptoms*: once they develop AVR is needed.
  If asx, HTN can be cautiously Rx'd (probably best w/ ACEI/ARB rather than diuretics).
  Statins have not been proven to ↓ progression.
- **AVR**
  Indicated in: **sx severe AS** (ie, stage D1); **asx severe AS + EF <50%** (stage C2);
  or asx severe (stage C1) *and* undergoing other cardiac surgery.
  Reasonable if:
  asx severe AS (stage C1) *but* either **sx or ↓ BP w/ exercise** (can *carefully*
  exercise asx AS to uncover sx, do *not* exercise sx AS) or **very severe**
  sx severe w/ low flow/∇ w/ low EF & response to dobuta (stage D2) or normal EF but AS felt to be cause of sx (stage D3)
  asx moderate AS (stage B) *and* undergoing cardiac surgery
- Transcatheter AoV replacement (TAVR, see below) indicated if surgical risk prohibitive or as
  reasonable alternative to surgery if high operative risk (STS predicted mortality 8–15%)
- Medical (if not AVR candidate or to temporize): careful diuresis prn, control HTN,
  maintain SR; digoxin if ↓ EF & HF or if AF; *avoid* venodilators (nitrates) & ⊖ inotropes
  (βB/CCB) if severe; avoid vigorous physical exertion once AS mod–severe;
  ? nitroprusside if p/w CHF & sev. AS, EF <35%, CI <2.2, & nl BP (*NEJM* 2003;348:1756)
- IABP: stabilization, bridge to surgery
- Balloon AoV valvotomy (BAV): 50% ↑ AVA & ↓ peak ∇, *but* 50% restenosis by 6–12 mo &
  ↑ risk of peri-PAV stroke/AR (*NEJM* 1988;319:125), ∴ bridge to AVR or palliation

TAVR (transcatheter AoV replacement)

- Catheter-based technique for replacing diseased AoV with bioprosthetic valve
- Valves: balloon-expandable (Edwards SAPIEN) or self-expanding (Medtronic CoreValve);
  balloon-expandable w/ less AR, less redo, less need for PPM (*JAMA* 2014;311:1503)
- Approaches: primarily retrograde via percutaneous transfemoral access; also retrograde
  via axillary artery or ascending aorta (via small sternotomy & aortotomy); alternatively
  transapical via direct LV apical puncture and antegrade implantation through small
  thoracotomy (if severe PAD or heavily calcified ascending Ao & arch)
- Periprocedural: local anesthesia w/ conscious sedation or general anesthesia; RV pacing
  (to decrease SV during deployment); TEE to guide placement
- Peri- & postprocedural complications: low CO, annular rupture or coronary occlusion
  (both rare), local vascular complications, paravalvular leaks & heart block (see below)
- ASA lifelong + clopidogrel × 6 mo
- Outcomes
  in nonoperative Pts vs med Rx: 44% ↓ mortality, but still ~20% annual mortality in TAVR
  group illustrating comorbidities in this population (*NEJM* 2012;366:1696; *JACC* 2014;63:1972)
  high-risk operative Pts vs surg AVR (*NEJM* 2012;366:1686 & 2014;370:1790)
  postop ≈ sx & hemodynamics
  mortality ≈ (balloon-expandable) or 26% ↓ (self-expanding) w/ TAVR vs surgery
  ↑ vasc complic; ↑ early risk of stroke/TIA w/ balloon-expandable
  heart block requiring PPM in ~20% w/ self-expanding; paravalvular leaks in ~7%
  prelim data in low-risk Pts shows lower mortality & stroke with TAVR (*JACC* 2015;65:2184)

AORTIC REGURGITATION (AR)

Etiology (*Circ* 2006;114:422)
- **Valve disease (43%)**
  rheumatic heart disease (usually mixed AS/AR and concomitant MV disease)
  bicuspid AoV: natural hx: $^1/_3$→ normal, $^1/_3$ → AS, $^1/_6$ → AR, $^1/_6$ → endocarditis → AR
  infective endocarditis
  valvulitis: RA, SLE; anorectics (fen/phen) & other serotoninergics (*NEJM* 2007;356:29,39), XRT
- **Root disease (57%)**
  HTN
  aortic aneurysm or dissection, annuloaortic ectasia, Marfan syndrome
  aortic inflammation: giant cell, Takayasu's, ankylosing spond., reactive arthritis, syphilis

Clinical manifestations
- Acute: sudden ↓ forward SV and ↑ LVEDP (noncompliant ventricle) → pulmonary edema
  ± hypotension and cardiogenic shock
- Chronic: clinically silent while LV dilates (to ↑ compliance to keep LVEDP low) more
  than it hypertrophies → chronic volume overload → LV decompensation → CHF
- Natural hx: *variable* progression (unlike AS, can be fast or slow); once decompensation
  begins, prognosis poor w/o AVR (mortality ~10%/y)

Physical exam

- **Early diastolic decrescendo murmur at LUSB** (RUSB if dilated Ao root); ↑ w/ sitting forward, expir, handgrip; severity of AR ∝ duration of murmur (except in acute and severe late); *Austin Flint murmur:* mid-to-late diastolic rumble at apex (AR jet interfering w/ mitral inflow)
- **Wide pulse pressure** due to ↑ stroke volume, hyper-dynamic pulse → many of classic signs (see table); pulse pressure narrows in late AR with ↓ LV fxn; bisferiens (twice-beating) arterial pulse
- PMI diffuse and laterally displaced; soft S_1 (early closure of MV); ± S_3 (≠ ↓ EF but rather just volume overload in AR)

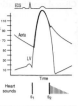

Classic Eponymous Signs in Chronic AR (South Med J 1981;74:459)	
Sign	**Description**
Corrigan's pulse	"water hammer" pulse (ie, rapid rise/fall or distention/collapse)
Hill's sign	(popliteal SBP – brachial SBP) >60 mmHg
Duroziez's sign	to-and-fro murmur heard over femoral artery w/ light compression
Pistol shot sounds	pistol shot sound heard over femoral artery
Traube's sound	double sound heard over femoral artery when compressed distally
de Musset's sign	head-bobbing with each heartbeat (low Se)
Müller's sign	systolic pulsations of the uvula
Quincke's pulses	subungual capillary pulsations (low Sp)

Diagnostic studies

- **ECG:** can see LVH, LAD, abnl repol; **CXR:** cardiomegaly ± ascending Ao dilatation
- **Echo:** severity of AR (in addition to parameters below, severe AR requires holodiastolic flow reversal in proximal abdominal Ao); LV size & fxn (chronic severe AR requires LV dilatation; LV dysfxn = EF <50% or LV end-syst. diam. [LVESD] >50 mm)
- **Cardiac MR** if TTE not sufficiently informative

Classification of Aortic Regurgitation				
Severity	**Regurg. fraction (%)**	**Jet width (% of LVOT)**	**ERO (cm²)**	**Angio***
Mild	<30	<25	<0.1	1+
Moderate	30–49	25–64	0.1–0.29	2+
Severe	≥50	≥65	≥0.3	3/4+

*1+ = incomplete LV opac.; 2+ = opac. < Ao root & clears 1 beat; 3+ = LV = Ao root opac.; LV > Ao root opac.

Treatment (Circ 2014;129:e521)

- **Acute decompensation** (consider ischemia and endocarditis as possible precipitants): *surgery* usually urgently needed for acute severe AR, which is poorly tolerated by LV IV afterload reduction (nitroprusside) and inotropic support (dobutamine) ± chronotropic support (↑ HR → ↓ diastole → ↓ time for regurgitation) pure vasoconstrictors and IABP contraindicated
- In chronic AR, management decisions based on *LV size and fxn* (and before sx occur)
- **Surgery** (AVR, replacement or repair if possible):
  severe and **sx** (if equivocal, consider stress test)
  asx and either **EF <50%** or **LV dilation** (LVESD >50 mm) or undergoing cardiac surg
- **Transcatheter AoV replacement (TAVR)** being explored (JACC 2013;61:1577)
- **Medical therapy:** **vasodilators** (nifedipine, ACEI/ARB, hydralazine) if severe AR w/ sx or LV dysfxn & Pt not operative candidate or to improve hemodynamics before AVR; no clear benefit on clinical outcomes or LV fxn when used to try to prolong compensation in asx severe AR w/ mild LV dilation & nl LV fxn (NEJM 2005;353:1342)

MITRAL REGURGITATION (MR)

Etiology (Lancet 2009;373:1382; NEJM 2010;363:156)

- **Primary** (degeneration of valve apparatus)
  leaflet abnl: myxomatous (MVP), endocarditis, calcific RHD, valvulitis (collagen-vascular disease), congenital, anorectic drugs, XRT
  chordae tendineae rupture: myxomatous, endocarditis, spontaneous, trauma
  papillary muscle dysfxn b/c of ischemia or rupture during MI [usu. posteromedial papillary m. (supplied by PDA only) vs anterolateral (suppl. by diags & OMs)]
- **Secondary (functional):** inferoapical papillary muscle displacement due to ischemic LV remodeling or other causes of DCM (JACC 2015;65:1231)

Clinical manifestations
- Acute: **pulmonary edema**, hypotension, cardiogenic shock (NEJM 2004;351:1627)
- Chronic: typically asx for yrs, then as LV fails → progressive DOE, fatigue, AF, PHT
- Prognosis: 5-y survival w/ medical therapy is 80% if asx, but only 45% if sx

Physical exam
- **High-pitched, blowing, holosystolic murmur at apex;**
  radiates to axilla; ± thrill; ↑ w/handgrip (Se 68%, Sp 92%),
  ↓ w/Valsalva (Se 93%) (NEJM 1988;318:1572)
  ant. leaflet abnl → post. jet heard at spine
  post. leaflet abnl → ant. jet heard at sternum
- ± diastolic rumble b/c ↑ flow across valve
- Lat. displ. hyperdynamic PMI, obscured S_1, widely split S_2
  (A_2 early b/c ↓ LV afterload, P_2 late if PHT); ± S_3
- Carotid upstroke brisk (vs diminished and delayed in AS)

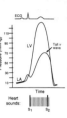

Diagnostic studies (NEJM 2005;352:875)
- ECG: may see LAE, LVH, ± atrial fibrillation
- CXR: dilated LA, dilated LV, ± pulmonary congestion
- **Echo:** MV anatomy (ie, etiol); MR severity: jet area (can underestimate eccentric jets), jet width at origin (vena contracta) or effective regurgitant orifice (ERO; predicts survival); LV fxn (EF should be *supranormal* if compensated, ∴ EF <60% w/ sev. MR = LV dysfxn); TEE if TTE inconclusive or pre/intraop to guide repair vs replace
- Cardiac MR if TTE not sufficiently informative
- **Cardiac cath:** prominent PCWP *c-v* waves (not spec. for MR), LVgram for MR severity & EF

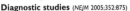

Classification of Primary Mitral Regurgitation					
Severity	**Regurg. fraction**	**Jet area** (% of LA)	**Jet width** (cm)	**ERO** (cm²)	**Angio***
Mild	<30%	<20	<0.3	<0.2	1+
Moderate	30–49%	20–40	0.3–0.69	0.2–0.39	2+
Severe†	≥50%	>40	≥0.70	≥0.40	3/4+

*1+ = LA clears w/ each beat; 2+ = LA does not clear, faintly opac. after several beats; 3+ = LA & LV opac. equal.
†For secondary MR, because ERO underestimated & likely progressive LV dysfxn, ERO ≥0.20 is severe

Treatment (Circ 2014;129:e521)
- Acute decompensation (consider ischemia and endocarditis as precipitants)
  IV afterload reduction (nitroprusside), ± inotropes (dobuta), IABP, avoid vasoconstrictors
  surgery usually needed for acute severe MR as prognosis poor w/o surgery (JAMA 2013;310:609)
- **Surgery** (repair [preferred if feasible] vs replacement w/ preservation of mitral apparatus)
  for **severe** primary MR
    indicated if **sx & EF >30%** or if **asx & either EF 30–60% or LV sys. diam. ≥40 mm**
    MV repair reasonable if asx & either EF >60% + LVESD <40 mm or new AF or PHT
    if AF, maze procedure or pulm vein isolation → ↓ AF recurrence, ∅ Δ stroke;
    consider for sx cntl or if planning no anticoag (NEJM 2015;372:1399)
  for **severe** secondary MR: consider if NYHA III-IV; replacement results in more durable correction than repair but no difference in clinical outcomes (NEJM 2014;370:23)
- In Pts undergoing CABG w/ mod–sev fxnal MR, annuloplasty ↓ MR but longer surgery, ↑ neurologic events, & no impact on fxnal status or mortality (NEJM 2014;371:2178)
- Percut. MV repair (Circ 2014;130:1712): edge-to-edge clip less effective than surgery but consider for sev. sx nonoperative Pt (NEJM 2011;364:1395); perc valve under study (JACC 2014;64:1814)
- Medical: ∅ clinical benefit in asx Pts; βB preserve LV fxn (JACC 2012;60:833); if sx but not operative candidate ↓ **preload** (↓ HF and MR by ↓ MV orifice): diuretics, nitrates (espec if ischemic/fxnal MR); if LV dysfxn: ACEI, βB, ± BiV pacing; maintain SR

MITRAL STENOSIS (MS)

Etiology (Lancet 2012;379:953)
- **Rheumatic heart disease** (RHD): *fusion of commissures* → "fish-mouth" valve from autoimmune rxn to β strep infxn; seen largely in developing world today
- **Mitral annular calcification** (MAC): encroachment upon leaflets → functional MS
- Congenital, infectious endocarditis w/ large lesion, myxoma near MV, thrombus
- Valvulitis (eg, SLE, amyloid, carcinoid) or infiltration (eg, mucopolysaccharidoses)

Clinical manifestations (Lancet 2009;374:1271)
- **Dyspnea and pulmonary edema** (if due to RHD, sx usually begin in 30s)
  precipitants: exercise, fever, anemia, volume overload (incl. pregnancy), tachycardia, AF
- **Atrial fibrillation:** onset often precipitates heart failure in Pts w/ MS
- **Embolic events:** commonly cerebral, espec in AF or endocarditis

- **Pulmonary:** hemoptysis, frequent bronchitis (due to congestion), PHT, RV failure
- **Ortner's syndrome:** hoarseness from LA compression of recurrent laryngeal nerve

Physical exam

- **Low-pitched mid-diastolic rumble at apex**
  w/ presystolic accentuation (if not in AF); best
  heard in L lat decubitus position during expi-
  ration, ↑ w/ exercise; severity proportional to
  duration (not intensity) of murmur

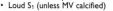
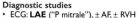

- **Opening snap** (high-pitched early diastolic
  sound at apex) from fused leaflet tips;
  MVA proportional to S_2–OS interval (tighter
  valve → ↑ LA pressure → shorter interval)
- Loud S_1 (unless MV calcified)

Diagnostic studies

- **ECG: LAE** ("P mitrale"), ± AF, ± RVH
- **CXR: dilated LA** (straightening of left heart border, double density on right, left mainstem bronchus elevation)
- **Echo:** estimate pressure gradient (∇), RVSP, valve area, valve echo score (0–16, based on leaflet mobility & thick., subvalvular thick., Ca^{++}); exer. TTE (to assess Δ RVSP and ∇) if sx & severity of MS at rest discrepant; TEE to assess for LA thrombus before PMV
- **Cardiac cath:** ∇ from simultaneous PCWP & LV pressures, calculated MVA; LA pressure tall *a* wave and blunted *y* descent; ↑ PA pressures

Classification of Mitral Stenosis				
Stage	**Mean ∇ (mmHg)**	**Pressure ½ time**	**MV area (cm²)**	**PA systolic (mmHg)**
Normal	0		4–6	<25
Mild-Mod	<5	100–149	1.6–2	<30
Severe	5–9	150–219	1.1–1.5	30–50
Very severe	≥10	≥220	≤1	>50

Treatment (*Circ* 2014;129:e521)

- Medical: Na restriction, cautious diuresis, βB, sx-limited physical stress
- Antibiotic Ppx recommended if h/o RHD w/ valvular disease for 10 y or until age 40
- Anticoag if: AF; prior embolism; LA thrombus; ? LA >55 mm or lg LA w/ spont contrast
- Mechanical intervention indicated if **heart failure sx w/ MVA ≤1.5;**
  reasonable if asx but very severe (MVA ≤1) and morphology favorable for PMBC;
  may consider PMBC if MVA >1.5 but hemodyn signif w/ exercise, or if asx but
  MVA ≤1.5 and new-onset AF
- **Percutaneous mitral balloon commissurotomy (PMBC):** preferred Rx if RHD;
  MVA doubles, ∇ ↓ by 50%; ≈ MVR if valve score <8, ≤ mild MR, ∅ AF or LA clot
- Surgical (MV repair if possible, o/w replacement): consider in sx Pts w/ MVA ≤1.5
  if PMV unavailable/contraindicated (mod. MR, LA clot), or valve morphology unsuitable
- Pregnancy: if NYHA class III/IV → PMV, o/w medical Rx w/ low-dose diuretic & βB

MITRAL VALVE PROLAPSE (MVP)

Definition and Etiology

- Billowing of MV leaflet ≥2 mm above mitral annulus in parasternal long axis echo view
- Leaflet redundancy from myxomatous proliferation of spongiosa of MV apparatus
- Idiopathic, familial and a/w connective tissue diseases (eg, Marfan's, Ehlers-Danlos)
- Prevalence 1–2.5% of gen. population, ♀ > ♂ (*NEJM* 1999;341:1), most common cause of MR

Clinical manifestations (usually asymptomatic)

- MR (from leaflet prolapse or ruptured chordae); infective endocarditis; embolic events
- Arrhythmias, rarely sudden cardiac death

Physical exam

- High-pitched, midsystolic click ± mid-to-late systolic murmur
- ↓ LV volume (standing) → click earlier; ↑ LV volume or afterload → click later, softer

Treatment

- Endocarditis prophylaxis no longer recommended (*Circ* 2007;116:1736)
- Aspirin or anticoagulation if prior neurologic event or atrial fibrillation

TRICUSPID REGURGITATION

- Primary etiol: rheumatic, CTD, radiation, IE, Ebstein's anomaly, carcinoid, tumors
- Fxnal etiol: RV and/or pulm HTN (may be 2° to L-sided dis.), RV dilation and/or infarct

- Assess based on severity TR, annular dilation, leaflet coaptation (JACC 2015;65:2331)
- Consider repair, annuloplasty or replacement for sx and severe TR (eg, ERO ≥ 0.40 cm²)

PROSTHETIC HEART VALVES

Mechanical (60%)
- Bileaflet (eg, St. Jude Medical); tilting disk; caged-ball
- Very durable (20–30 y), but thrombogenic and ∴ require anticoagulation
  consider if age <~60 y or if anticoagulation already indicated (JACC 2010;55:2413)

Bioprosthetic (40%)
- Bovine pericardial or porcine heterograft (eg, Carpentier-Edwards), homograft
- Less durable, but min. thrombogenic; consider if >~70 y, lifespan <20 y or ∅ anticoag
- If 50–69 y, 2× reop but ½ bleeding or stroke vs mech (JAMA 2014;312:1323 & 2015;313:1435)

Physical exam
- Normal: **crisp sounds**, ± soft murmur during forward flow (normal to have small ▽)
- Abnormal: regurgitant murmurs, absent mechanical valve closure sounds

Anticoagulation & antiplatelet therapy (Circ 2014;129:e521)
- Assess for high-risk features: prior thromboembolism, AF, EF<30–35%, hypercoagulable
- **Warfarin:** low-risk mech AVR: INR 2–3
  mech MVR or high-risk mech AVR: INR 2.5–3.5
  high-risk bioprosthetic: INR 2–3; for 1st 3 mo, reasonable in low-risk MVR, consider in
  low-risk AVR
- **ASA** (75–100 mg) for all prosthetic valves; avoid adding to warfarin if h/o GIB, uncontrolled
  HTN, erratic INR or >80 y
- If thrombosis, ↑ intensity (eg, INR 2–3 → 2.5-3.5; 2.5–3.5 → 3.5-4.5; add ASA if not on)

Periprocedural "Bridging" of Anticoagulation in Pts with Mechanical Valve(s)	
AVR w/o risk factors	d/c warfarin 2–4 before surg; restart 12–24 h after surg
MVR or AVR w/ risk factors	Preop: d/c warfarin, start UFH when INR <2
	4–6 h preop: d/c UFH; postop: restart UFH & warfarin ASAP

Procedures include noncardiac surgery, invasive procedures, and major dental work

Correction of overanticoagulation (Circ 2014;129:e521)
- Risk from major bleeding must be weighed against risk of valve thrombosis
- Not bleeding: if INR 5–10, withhold warfarin; if INR >10 also give vit K 1–2.5 mg PO
- Bleeding: FFP or PCC ± low-dose (1 mg) vit K IV

Endocarditis prophylaxis: for all prosthetic valves (see "Endocarditis")

Complications
- Structural failure (r/o endocarditis); mechanical valves: rare except for Bjork-Shiley; bio-
  prosth: up to 30% rate w/in 10–15 y, mitral > aortic; consider TAVR (JAMA 2014;312:162)
- Paravalvular leak (r/o endocarditis); small central jet of regurg is normal in mech. valves
- Obstruction from thrombosis or pannus ingrowth: ✓ TTE, TEE, and/or fluoroscopy if ? clot
  significantly sx pannus ingrowth: remove w/ surgery
  thrombosis: surgery if L-sided valve & either severe sx or lg (? ≥0.8 cm) thrombus;
  lytic often ineffective for L-sided thrombosis 12–15% risk of stroke; consider
  UFH ± lytic (? low-dose tPA via slow infusion, JACC CV Imaging 2013;6:206) if mild sx &
  small clot burden or poor surg candidate; lytic reasonable for R-sided
- Infective endocarditis ± valvular abscess and conduction system dis. (see "Endocarditis")
- Embolization (r/o endocarditis); risk ~1%/y w/ warfarin (vs 2% w/ ASA, or 4% w/o meds)
  mech MVR 2× risk of embolic events vs mech AVR (Circ 1994;89:635)
- Bleeding (from anticoag), hemolysis (espec w/ caged-ball valves or paravalvular leak)

HEART VALVES (superior view, JAMA 1976;235:1603)

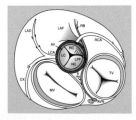

AV = aortic valve
AVN = AV node
B His = bundle of His
CS = coronary sinus
Cx = circumflex artery
LAD = left anterior descending artery
LAF = left anterior fascicle
LCA = left coronary artery
LPF = left posterior fascicle
MV = mitral valve
RB = right bundle
RC/LC/NC = right/left/noncoronary cusp
RCA = right coronary artery
TV = tricuspid valve

CARDIOPULMONARY EXERCISE TESTING

Background, rationale, and measurements performed (Circ 2010;122:191)
- In exercise, to meet metabolic demands of active cells, need to ↑ effective ventilation, ↑ cardiac output, and ↓ pulmonary & systemic vascular resistance, ↑ O_2 extraction
- Dyspnea due to insufficient supply to or impaired uptake of O_2 by skeletal muscle
- Ddx of dyspnea:
    - impaired external respiration (ventilation & pulmonary gas exchange)
    - impaired circulatory system (transport of O_2 and CO_2)
    - impaired internal respiration (peripheral capillary gas exchange and O_2 utilization)
- Cardiorespiratory fitness predicts morbidity & mortality
- CPET is an individualized incremental exercise test that combines
    - traditional cardiac stress test parameters: ECG, heart rate, BP
    - quantification of O_2 consumption (VO_2), CO_2 production (VO_2), minute ventilation (V_E)
    - if invasive (radial artery & PA cath): RAP, PAP, & PCWP; arterial & mixed venous sats
    - can be coupled with cardiac imaging (eg, radionuclide ventriculography, TTE)
- Well tolerated even w/ advanced disease, 0.16% adverse event rate (Circ 2012;126:2465)

Indications for CPET
- Diagnose etiology of exercise intolerance or dyspnea by defining organ system limiting gas exchange (heart, pulm mechanical, pulm vasculature, muscles/mitochondria)
- Grade severity of advanced heart and lung diseases and predict prognosis
    - Prioritize Pts for heart/lung transplantation, mechanical support:
        - Heart transplant candidacy: peak VO_2 <14 ml/kg/min, <12 on βB, ± <50% predicted
        - LVAD candidacy <12 ml/kg/min (NEJM 2001;345:1445)
    - Determine whether to intervene on valvular disease, shunts/congenital heart disease
- To objectively measure responses to interventions (clinical trials, disability, rehabilitation)

Clinical relevance of measurement patterns
- RER (respiratory exchange ratio) = VCO_2/VO_2, indicator of volitional effort independent of chronotropic response (goal >1.05)
- V_E/MVV (max voluntary vent): >70–80% indicates encroachment on pulm mechanical limit
- Peak VO_2: max aerobic capacity at peak exercise; indicator of cardiorespiratory fitness measured with metabolic cart but also represented by the Fick equation:
    - VO_2 = (heart rate × stroke volume) × [(arterial − mixed venous) O_2 content]
- VAT (ventilatory anaerobic threshold): % of peak predicted VO_2 at which O_2 supply inadequate → anaerobic metabolism (normal value >40%); indep. of volitional effort, highly reproducible, and occurs at activity levels often assoc. w/ daily living. Low VAT reflects impaired O_2 delivery ± utilization but does not localize organ system responsible. In HFrEF, VAT<11 ml/kg/min assoc w/ 5× ↑ in 6-mo mortality (Circ 2002;106:3079).
- V_E/VCO_2 slope: ventilation required to exchange 1 L/min of CO_2
    - in addition, V_E/VCO_2 slope = constant / [P_aCO_2 × (1 − V_d/V_t)]
    - high level (>36) especially seen in pulm vascular and/or RV dysfunction, where V/Q mismatch & ↓ pulm perfusion → ↑ V_d/V_t, and ↑ ventilatory drive → ↓ P_aCO_2
    - high levels also indicate poor prognosis (Circ 2007;115:2410; Circ HF 2008;1:227)
- Exercise oscillatory vent: periodic breathing that reflects circul. delay (ie, low CO) relative to metab needs during exercise; assoc w/ 3× ↑ mort (JACC 2010;55:1814; Circ 2011;124:1442)
- mPAP/CO slope (serial measurements during exercise define the pulm artery pressure response to increased blood flow through the pulmonary circulation during exercise): mPAP = TPG + LAP
    - mPAP/CO slope >3 indicates either abnl pulm vascular response to exercise or upstream transmission of high LAP (Circ 2013;128:1470), with TPG/CO (ie, PVR) that fails to fall and remains >1.5 indicative of pulmonary vascular dysfunction and PCWP/CO slope >2 indicative of left-sided failure
- DPG (diastolic pulmonary gradient) = PAD − LAP; DPG >5–7 indicates pulm vasc disease and may be preferable to TPG (mPAP − LAP) for pulm vasc disease diagnosis b/c it is not significantly influenced by ΔLAP and CO (Chest 2013;143:758)

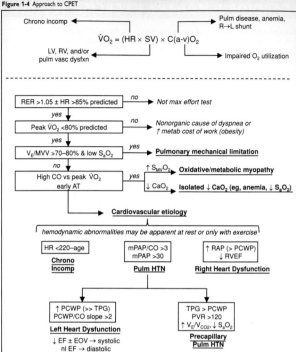

Figure 1-4 Approach to CPET

Chrono incomp ◄─────────────┐   ┌────────► Pulm disease, anemia, R→L shunt

$$\dot{V}O_2 = (HR \times SV) \times C(a\text{-}v)O_2$$

LV, RV, and/or pulm vasc dysfxn ◄───┘   └────► Impaired O_2 utilization

- -

RER >1.05 ± HR >85% predicted ──*no*──► *Not max effort test*

↓ *yes*

Peak $\dot{V}O_2$ <80% predicted ──*no*──► *Nonorganic cause of dyspnea or ↑ metab cost of work (obesity)*

↓ *yes*

V_E/MVV >70–80% & low S_aO_2 ──*yes*──► **Pulmonary mechanical limitation**

↓ *no*

High CO vs peak $\dot{V}O_2$ early AT ──*yes*──► ↑ $S_{M_VO_2}$ ► **Oxidative/metabolic myopathy**

↓ CaO_2 ► **Isolated ↓ CaO_2 (eg, anemia, ↓ S_aO_2)**

└────────► **Cardiovascular etiology**

┌─ *hemodynamic abnormalities may be apparent at rest or only with exercise* ─

HR <220–age
Chrono Incomp

mPAP/CO >3
mPAP >30
Pulm HTN

↑ RAP (> PCWP)
↓ RVEF
Right Heart Dysfunction

↑ PCWP (>> TPG)
PCWP/CO slope >2
Left Heart Dysfunction
↓ EF ± EOV → systolic
nl EF → diastolic

TPG > PCWP
PVR >120
↑ V_E/V_{CO_2}, ↓ S_aO_2
Precapillary Pulm HTN

PERICARDIAL DISEASE

GENERAL PRINCIPLES

Anatomy
• 2-layered (parietal & visceral) tissue sac surrounding heart & proximal great vessels

Disease states
• Inflammation (w/ or w/o fluid accumulation) → pericarditis
• Fluid accumulation → effusion ± tamponade
• Decrease in compliance (sequela of inflammation) → constrictive pericarditis
• Tamponade and constriction characterized by increased ventricular interdependence

PERICARDITIS AND PERICARDIAL EFFUSION

Etiologies of Acute Pericarditis (Lancet 2004;363:717; Curr Probl Cardiol 2012;37:75)	
Idiopathic (~90%)	Most presumed to be undiagnosed viral etiologies
Infectious (<5% can be confirmed infectious)	Viral: Coxsackie, echo, adeno, EBV, VZV, HIV, influenza Bacterial (from endocarditis, pneumonia or s/p cardiac surgery): S. pneumococcus, N. meningitidis, S. aureus, Borrelia (Lyme); TB Fungal: Histo, Coccidio, Candida; Parasitic: Entamoeba, Echino
Neoplastic (<10%)	Common: metastatic (lung, breast, lymphoma, leukemia, RCC) Rare: primary cardiac & serosal tumors (mesothelioma)
Autoimmune	Connective tissue diseases: SLE, RA, scleroderma, Sjögren's Vasculitides: PAN, Churg-Strauss, Wegener's Drug-induced: procainamide, hydralazine, INH, CsA
Uremia	~5–13% of Pts prior to HD; ~20% occurrence in chronic HD Pts
Cardiovascular	Acute STEMI, late post-MI (Dressler's syndrome), but both rare in modern era; proximal AoD; chest trauma/postpericardiotomy
Radiation	>40 Gy to mediastinum; acute or delayed; may be transudative
Effusions w/o pericarditis	HF, cirrhosis, nephrotic syndrome, hypothyroidism, amyloidosis Transudative

Clinical manifestations (NEJM 2014;371:2410)
• **Pericarditis:** retrosternal chest pain that is pleuritic, positional (↓ by sitting forward), radiates to trapezius; may be absent in TB, neoplastic, post-XRT and uremic pericarditis; ± fever; ± s/s of systemic etiologies
• **Effusion:** ranges from asx to tamponade (see below)

Physical exam
• **Pericarditis:** multiphasic **friction rub** best heard at LLSB w/ diaphragm of stethoscope. Notoriously variable and evanescent leathery sound w/ up to 3 components: atrial contraction, ventricular contraction, ventricular relaxation (NEJM 2012;367:e20).
• **Effusion:** distant heart sounds, dullness over left posterior lung field due to compressive atelectasis from pericardial effusion (Ewart's sign)

Diagnostic studies (EHJ 2004;25:587; Circ 2006;113:1622 & 2010;121:916)
• **ECG:** may show diffuse STE (concave up) & PR depression (except in aVR: ST ↓ & PR ↑), TWI; classically and in contrast to STEMI, TWI do not occur until STs normalize
Stages: (I) STE & PR ↓; (II) ST & PR normalize; (III) TWI; (IV) Tw normalize
ECG may show evidence of large effusion w/ low voltage & electrical alternans (beat-to-beat Δ in QRS amplitude and/or axis due to swinging heart)
• **CXR:** if large effusion (>250 mL of fluid) → ↑ cardiac silhouette w/ "water-bottle" heart and epicardial halo
• **Echocardiogram:** presence, size, & location of effusion; presence of tamponade physiology; pericarditis itself w/o spec. abnl (∴ echo can be nl), although can see pericardial stranding (fibrin or tumor); can also detect LV/RV dysfxn (myocarditis ?)
• **CT** will reveal pericardial effusions, often appearing larger than on echocardiography
• **CK-MB** or troponin (⊕ in ~30%, JACC 2003;42:2144) if myopericarditis. Consider CRP/ESR.

Workup for effusion
• r/o infxn: usually apparent from Hx & CXR; ? value of ✓ acute and convalescent serologies
• r/o noninfectious etiologies: BUN, Cr, ANA, RF, HIV, screen for common malignancies
• Pericardiocentesis if suspect infxn or malignancy or large effusion (>2 cm) or recurrent
✓ cell counts, TP, LDH, glc, Gram stain & Cx, AFB, cytology
ADA, PCR for MTb, and specific tumor markers as indicated by clinical suspicion
"exudate" criteria: TP >3 g/dL, TP$_{eff}$/TP$_{serum}$ >0.5, LDH$_{eff}$/LDH$_{serum}$ >0.6 or glc <60 mg/dL
high Se (~90%) but very low Sp (~20%); overall low utility (Chest 1997;111:1213)
• Pericardial bx if suspicion remains for malignancy or TB

Treatment of pericarditis (Circ 2013;127:1723)

- High-dose **NSAID** (eg, ibuprofen 600–800 mg tid) or ASA (eg, 650–1000 mg tid) × 7–14 d then taper over wks; ASA preferred over NSAID in acute MI; consider PPI to ↓ risk of GIB
- Add **colchicine** 0.5 mg bid (qd if ≤70 kg) × 3 mo; ↓ risk of refractory or recurrent pericarditis by 50% (NEJM 2013;369:1522)
- Steroids (usually systemic; occ. intrapericardial) only for systemic rheum or autoimmune disorder, uremic, preg., contraindication to NSAID, or refractory idiopathic dis. Systemic steroids appear to ↑ rate of pericarditis recurrence (Circ 2008;118:667).
- Avoid anticoagulants (although no convincing data that ↑ risk of hemorrhage/tamponade)
- Infectious effusion → pericardial drainage (preferably surgically) + systemic antibiotics
- Acute idiopathic effusion self-limited in 70–90% of cases
- Recurrent pericarditis (Circ 2007;115:2739)
  risk factors: subacute, lg effusion/tamponade, T >38°C, lack of NSAID response after 7 d treatment: colchicine 0.5 mg bid × 6 mo (Annals 2011;155:409 & Lancet 2014;383:2232)
- Recurrent effusion: consider pericardial window (percutaneous vs surgical)

PERICARDIAL TAMPONADE

Etiology
- Any cause of pericarditis but espec **malignancy, uremia, idiopathic**, proximal aortic dissection with rupture, myocardial rupture
- Rapidly accumulating effusions most likely to cause tamponade as no time for pericardium to stretch (eg, to ↑ compliance) and accommodate ↑ intrapericardial fluid volume

Pathophysiology (NEJM 2003;349:684)
- ↑ intrapericardial pressure, compression of heart chambers, ↓ venous return → ↓ CO
- Diastolic pressures ↑ & equalize in all cardiac chambers → minimal flow of blood from RA to RV when TV opens → blunted y descent
- ↑ ventricular interdependence → pulsus paradoxus (pathologic exaggeration of nl physio) Inspiration → ↓ intrapericardial & RA pressures → ↑ venous return → ↑ RV size → septal shift to left. Also, ↑ pulmonary vascular compliance → ↓ pulm venous return. Result is ↓ LV filling → ↓ **LV stroke volume** & blood pressure.

Clinical manifestations
- **Cardiogenic shock** (hypotension, fatigue) **without pulmonary edema**
- Dyspnea (seen in ~85%) may be due to ↑ respiratory drive to augment venous return

Physical exam (JAMA 2007;297:1810)
- **Beck's triad** (present in minority of cases): **distant heart sounds, ↑ JVP, hypotension**
- ↑ JVP (76%) w/ blunted y descent
- Reflex tachycardia (77%), hypotension (26%; occasionally hypertensive), cool extremities
- **Pulsus paradoxus** (Se 82%, Sp 70%) = ↓ SBP ≥10 mmHg during inspiration
  ⊕ LR 3.3 (5.9 if pulsus >12), ⊖ LR 0.03
  Ddx = PE, hypovolemia, severe COPD, constriction (~⅓), RV infarct
  Can be absent if pre-existing ↑ LVEDP, arrhythmia, severe AI, ASD, regional tamponade
- Distant heart sounds (28%), ± pericardial friction rub (30%)
- Tachypnea but clear lungs

Diagnostic studies
- ECG: ↓ voltage (seen in 42%), electrical alternans (20%), ± signs of pericarditis
- CXR: ↑ cardiac silhouette (89%)
- **Echocardiogram**: ⊕ **effusion**, IVC plethora, **septal shift** with inspiration **diastolic collapse** of RA (Se 85%, Sp 80%) and/or RV (Se <80%, Sp 90%) **respirophasic ∆'s in transvalvular velocities** (↑ across TV & ↓ across MV w/ inspir.) postsurgical tamponade may be localized and not easily visible
- Cardiac cath (right heart and pericardial): elevation (15–30 mmHg) and equalization of intrapericardial and diastolic pressures (RA, RV, PCWP), blunted y descent in RA ↑ in stroke volume postpericardiocentesis = ultimate proof of tamponade if RA pressure remains elevated after drainage, may have effusive-constrictive disease (NEJM 2004;350:469) or myocardial dysfxn (eg, from concomitant myocarditis)

Treatment
- Volume (but be careful as overfilling can worsen tamponade) and ⊕ inotropes (avoid βB)
- Avoid vasoconstrictors as will ↓ stroke volume & potentially ↓ HR
- **Pericardiocentesis** (except if due to aortic or myocardial rupture, in which case consider removing just enough fluid to reverse PEA en route to emergent surgery)

CONSTRICTIVE PERICARDITIS

Etiology (Circ 2011;124:1270)
- Any cause of pericarditis (~1–2% incidence overall after acute pericarditis)
- Highest risk w/ **TB, bacterial**, neoplastic, connective tissue, postcardiac surgery
- **Viral/idiopathic**, as most common cause of pericarditis, also account for signif proportion

Pathophysiology
- Adhesion of visceral and parietal pericardial layers → rigid pericardium that limits diastolic filling of ventricles → ↑ systemic venous pressures
- Venous return is limited only after early diastolic filling phase; ∴ rapid ↓ in RA pressure with atrial relaxation and opening of tricuspid valve and *prominent x and y descents*
- Kussmaul sign: JVP does not decrease with inspiration (↑ venous return with inspiration, but negative intrathoracic pressure not transmitted to heart because of rigid pericardium)

Clinical manifestations (NEJM 2011;364:1350)
- Right-sided > left-sided heart failure (systemic congestion > pulmonary congestion)

Physical exam
- ↑ **JVP** with **prominent y descent, ⊕ Kussmaul sign** (Ddx: tricuspid stenosis, acute cor pulmonale, RV failure and RV infarct, RCMP)
- Hepatosplenomegaly, ascites, peripheral edema. Consider on Ddx of idiopathic cirrhosis.
- PMI usually not palpable, **pericardial knock**, usually no pulsus paradoxus

Diagnostic studies
- ECG: nonspecific, AF common (up to 33%) in advanced cases
- CXR: calcification (MTb most common), espec in lateral view (although not specific)
- Echocardiogram: ± thickened pericardium, "septal bounce" = abrupt displacement of septum during rapid filling in early diastole
- Cardiac catheterization: atria w/ **Ms** or **Ws** (prominent x and y descents)
  ventricles: **dip-and-plateau** or **square-root sign** (rapid ↓ pressure at onset of diastole, rapid ↑ to early plateau)
  discordance between LV & RV pressure peaks during respiratory cycle (Circ 1996;93:2007)
- CT or MRI: thickened pericardium (>4 mm; Se ~80%) w/ tethering (Circ 2011;123:e418)

Treatment
- Diuresis for intravascular volume overload; surgical pericardiectomy in advanced cases
- ? MRI able to predict reversibility with anti-inflammatory agents (Circ 2011;124:1830)

Constrictive Pericarditis vs Restrictive Cardiomyopathy		
Evaluation	**Constrictive pericarditis**	**Restrictive cardiomyopathy**
Physical exam	⊕ Kussmaul sign Absent PMI ⊕ Pericardial knock	± Kussmaul sign Powerful PMI, ± S_3 and S_4 **± Murmurs of MR, TR**
ECG	± Low voltage	Low voltage if infiltrative myopathy **± Conduction abnormalities**
Echocardiogram	**Respirophasic variation** (25–40%): inspir. → ↑ flow across TV and ↓ flow across MV E' (tissue velocity) nl/↑ (>12) **Expir.** hepatic vein flow reversal **Septal bounce** during early diastole Normal wall thickness	<10% respirophasic variation Slower peak filling rate Longer time to peak filling rate **E'** ↓ (<8 cm/sec) **Inspir.** hepatic vein flow reversal **Biatrial enlargement** ± ↑ wall thickness
CT/MRI	**Thickened pericardium**	Normal pericardium
NT-proBNP	Variable	Typically ↑/↑↑ (JACC 2005;45:1900)
Cardiac catheterization	Prominent x and y descents Dip-and-plateau sign	
	LVEDP = RVEDP RVSP <55 mmHg (Se 90%, Sp 29%) RVEDP >$^{1}/_{3}$ RVSP (Se 93%, Sp 46%) **Discordance** of LV & RV pressure peaks during respiratory cycle **Systolic area index** (ratio of RV to LV pressure–time area in inspir vs expir) >1.1 (Se 97%, Sp 100%)	**LVEDP > RVEDP** (esp. w/ vol.) RVSP >55 mmHg RVEDP <$^{1}/_{3}$ RVSP Concordance of LV & RV pressure peaks during respiratory cycle Systolic area index ≤1.1 (JACC 2008;51:315)
Endomyocardial biopsy	Usually normal	**± Specific etiology of RCMP** (fibrosis, infiltration, hypertrophy)

HYPERTENSION

Classification		
Category	**Systolic (mmHg)**	**Diastolic (mmHg)**
Normal	<120	<80
Pre-HTN	120–139	80–89
Stage 1 HTN	140–159	90–99
Stage 2 HTN	≥160	≥100

Average ≥2 measurements >1–2 min apart. Confirm stage 1 w/in 1-4 wk; can Rx stage 2 immediately. ✓ q2y (if nl) or yearly (if pre-HTN). (J Clin HTN 2014;16:14)

Ambulatory Thresholds		
Setting	**Systolic (mmHg)**	**Diastolic (mmHg)**
24-hr average	135	85
Day* (awake)	140	90
Night (asleep)	125	75

*Threshold of hypertension for home readings should be same as daytime ambulatory

Epidemiology (Circulation 2012;125:e2)
- Prevalence 33.5% in U.S. adults; >75 million affected (prevalence equal for men and women, highest in African American adults at 44%)
- ↑ Age → ↓ arterial compliance → systolic HTN
- Only 48% of patients with dx of HTN have adequate BP control

Etiologies
- **Essential** (95%): onset 25–55 y; ⊕ FHx. Unclear mechanism but ? additive microvasc renal injury over time w/ contribution of hyperactive sympathetics (NEJM 2002;346:913). Both genetic (Nature 2011;478:103) & environmental risk factors (Na, obesity, inactivity) Blacks more likely to be salt sensitive and have less activation of renin-angiotensin system, explaining preference for thiazides & CCB over ACEI or ARB
- **Secondary:** Consider if Pt <20 or >50 y or if sudden onset, severe, refractory HTN

Secondary Causes of Hypertension			
Diseases		**Suggestive findings**	**Initial workup**
RENAL	**Renal parenchymal** (2–3%)	h/o DM, polycystic kidney disease, glomerulonephritis	CrCl, albuminuria See "Renal Failure"
	Renovascular (1–2%, qv) Athero (90%) FMD (10%, women) PAN, scleroderma	ARF induced by ACEI/ARB Recurrent flash pulm edema Renal bruit; hypokalemia (NEJM 2009;361:1972)	MRA (>90% Se & Sp, less for FMD), CTA, duplex U/S, angio, plasma renin (low Sp)
ENDO	**Hyperaldo or Cushing's** (1–5%)	Hypokalemia Metabolic alkalosis	See "Adrenal Disorders"
	Pheochromocytoma (<1%)	Paroxysmal HTN, H/A, palp.	
	Myxedema (<1%)	See "Thyroid Disorders"	TFTs
	Hypercalcemia (<1%)	Polyuria, dehydration, ∆ MS	iCa
OTHER	**Obstructive sleep apnea** (qv)		
	Medications: OCP, steroids, licorice; NSAIDs (espec COX-2); Epo; cyclosporine		
	Aortic coarctation: ↓ LE pulses, systolic murmur; radial-femoral delay; abnl TTE, CXR		
	Polycythemia vera: ↑ Hct		

Standard workup (J Clin HTN 2014;16:14)
- Goals: (1) identify CV risk factors or other diseases that would modify prognosis or Rx; (2) reveal 2° causes of hypertension; (3) assess for target-organ damage
- History: CAD, HF, TIA/CVA, PAD, DM, renal insufficiency, sleep apnea, preeclampsia; ⊕ FHx for HTN; diet, Na intake, smoking, alcohol, prescription and OTC meds, OCP
- Physical exam: ✓ **BP in both arms**; funduscopic exam; BMI & waist circumference; cardiac (LVH, murmurs) including signs of HF, vascular (bruits, radial-femoral delay); abdominal (masses or bruits); neuro exam
- Testing: K, BUN, Cr, Ca, glc, Hct, U/A, lipids, TSH, urinary albumin:creatinine (if ↑ Cr, DM, or peripheral edema), ? renin, ECG (for LVH), CXR, TTE (for valve abnl, LVH)
- Ambulatory BP monitoring (ABPM): predictive of CV risk and ↑ Se & Sp for dx of HTN vs office BP (HTN 2005;46:156). Consider for suspected episodic or white coat HTN, resistant HTN, HoTN sx on meds, or suspected autonomic dysfxn. Rec by some guidelines to confirm HTN dx, so utilization may expand (BMJ 2011;342:d3621 & 343:d4891).

Complications of HTN
- Each ↑ 20 mmHg SBP or 10 mmHg DBP → 2× ↑ CV complications (Lancet 2002;360:1903)
- Neurologic: **TIA/CVA**, ruptured aneurysms, vascular dementia

- Retinopathy: stage I = arteriolar narrowing; II = copper wiring, AV nicking;
  III = hemorrhages and exudates; IV = papilledema
- Cardiac: **CAD, LVH, HF, AF**
- Vascular: aortic dissection, aortic aneurysm (HTN = key risk factor for aneurysms)
- Renal: proteinuria, **renal failure**

Treatment *(JAMA 2014;311:507; J Clin HTN 2014;16:14; JACC 2015;65:1998)*
- Goal: in general, **<140/90 mmHg**
  In elderly: data sparser, but benefit, albeit w/ less strict BP target *(NEJM 2008;358:1887);*
    thus, consider <150/90 mmHg if either (a) ≥80 y and w/o DM or CKD (ASH/ISH rec),
    or (b) ≥60 y (but no need to downtitrate if <140/90 & tolerating meds) (JNC 8 rec)
  In Pts w/ prior MI or stroke: reasonable to consider <130/80 *(HTN 2015;65:1372)*
  In Pts w/ DM and/or CKD: prior targets of <130/80 not supported by data (and
    harm if target <120; NEJM 2010;362:1575), but may consider if CKD & albuminuria
    for renal protection (ASH/ISH rec based on NEJM 1994;330:877)
- *Treatment results in 50% ↓ HF, 40% ↓ stroke, 20–25% ↓ MI (Lancet 2014;384:591)*
- **Lifestyle modifications** (each ↓ SBP ~5 mmHg)
  weight loss: goal BMI 18.5–24.9; aerobic exercise: ≥30 min exercise/d, ≥5 d/wk
  diet: rich in fruits & vegetables, low in saturated & total fat (DASH, NEJM 2001;344:3)
  sodium restriction: ≤2.4 g/d and ideally ≤1.5 g/d *(NEJM 2010;362:2102)*
  maintain adequate potassium intake through diet counseling (~120 mEq of dietary
    potassium) if no predisposition to hyperkalemia *(NEJM 2007;356:1966)*
  limit alcohol consumption: ≤2 drinks/d in ♂; ≤1 drink/d in ♀ & lighter-wt Pts
  avoid exacerbating exposures (eg, NSAID use)
- **Pharmacologic options** for HTN or pre-HTN w/ comorbidity (nb, pre-HTN w/o
    DM, CKD, CV disease, or other end organ dysfunction treated w/ lifestyle alone)
  Pre-HTN: ARB prevents onset of HTN, no ↓ in clinical events (NEJM 2006;354:1685)
  HTN: *choice of therapy controversial, concomitant disease and stage may help guide Rx*
  uncomplicated: CCB, ARB or ACEI, or thiazide (chlorthalidone preferred) are
    1st line (NEJM 2009;361:2153); βB not 1st line (Lancet 2005;366:1545).
    For non-black Pts <60 y: reasonable to start w/ ARB or ACEI, then add CCB or thiazide
      if needed, and then add remaining class if still needed
    For black, elderly, and ? obese Pts (all of whom more likely to be salt sensitive):
      reasonable to start with CCB or thiazide, then add either the other 1st choice class
      or ARB or ACEI if needed, and then all 3 classes if still needed
  +CAD (Circ 2015;131:e435): ACEI or ARB (NEJM 2008;358:1547); ACEI+CCB superior to
    ACEI+thiazide (NEJM 2008;359:2417) or βB (NEJM 2003;366:895); may require βB
    and/or nitrates for anginal relief; if h/o MI, add ± ACEI/ARB ± aldo antag (see "ACS")
  +HF: ACEI/ARB, βB, diuretics, aldosterone antagonist (see "Heart Failure")
  +2° stroke prevention: ACEI (Lancet 2001;358:1033); ? ARB (NEJM 2008;359:1225)
  +diabetes mellitus: ACEI or ARB; can also consider thiazide or CCB
  +chronic kidney disease: ACEI or ARB (NEJM 1993;329:1456 & 2001;345:831 & 861)
- **Tailoring therapy**
  lifestyle Δs typically complementary rather than alternative to drug Rx [although if
    low risk (stage 1, no end-organ damage or risk factors), could start with lifestyle]
  if stage 1, start w/ monoRx; if stage 2, consider starting w/ combo (eg, ACEI + CCB;
    NEJM 2008;359:2417), as most will require ≥2 drugs
  typically start drug at ½ maximal dose; after 2–3 wk either titrate up or add new drug

Resistant hypertension *(JAMA 2014;311:2216)*
- BP > goal on ≥3 drugs incl diuretic, ~12–13% of hypertensive population (HTN 2011;57:1105)
- Differentiate between true & *pseudoresistance,* w/ latter due to:
  inaccurate measurement or use of wrong cuff size
  poor dietary compliance (Na/K intake, can assess w/ 24-hr urine for Na, K and Cr)
  suboptimal med dosing (eg, <50% of max dose) or poor med compliance
  volume expansion (inadequate diuretic dosing)
  white coat HTN (consider ABPM)
  2° causes or external drivers (eg, OSA, steroids, NSAIDS, alcohol) (Lancet 2010;376:1903)
- True resistance = uncontrolled BP confirmed by ABPM despite compliance w/ optim. doses
- Treatment considerations:
  Persistent ↑ volume may contribute even if on standard HCTZ (Archives 2008;168:1159).
  Effective diuretic dosing required for most to achieve control (HTN 2002;39:982).
  Chlorthalidone over HCTZ (if renal function preserved). Loop diuretic favored over
    thiazide for initial Rx if eGFR <30; however, adding thiazide to loop can ↑ diuresis if
    insufficient response to loop alone.
  Adding aldosterone antagonist (if renal function preserved) (PATHWAY-2, ESC 2015)
  Adding β-blocker (particularly vasodilating ones such as labetalol, carvedilol, or
    nebivolol), centrally acting agent, α-blocker, or direct vasodilator

Other Rx under investigation: renal denervation (see below); carotid baroreceptor stimulation; central AV anastomosis ↓ SBP by −23 mmHg (*Lancet* 2015;385:1634)
- **Renal denervation:** catheter-based RF ablation of renal nerves modifying sympathetic outflow. Had appeared beneficial in unblinded and/or uncontrolled studies, but no effect on BP in controlled trial, so not currently an option in routine care (*NEJM* 2014;370:1393).

Special situations
- **Secondary causes**
  Renovascular (qv)
  Renal parenchymal disease: salt and fluid restriction, ± diuretics
  Endocrine etiologies: see "Adrenal Disorders"
- **Pregnancy:** methyldopa, labetalol, nifedipine, hydralazine; avoid diuretics; ∅ ACEI/ARB

HYPERTENSIVE CRISES

- **Hypertensive emergency:** ↑ BP → acute target-organ ischemia and damage
  neurologic: encephalopathy (insidious onset of headache, nausea, vomiting, confusion), hemorrhagic or ischemic stroke, papilledema
  cardiac: ACS, HF/pulmonary edema, aortic dissection
  renal: proteinuria, hematuria, acute renal failure; scleroderma renal crisis
  microangiopathic hemolytic anemia; preeclampsia-eclampsia
- **Hypertensive urgency (severe asymptomatic HTN):** SBP >180 or DBP >120 (?110) w/ minimal or no target-organ damage

Precipitants
- Progression of essential HTN ± medical noncompliance (espec clonidine) or Δ in diet
- Progression of renovascular disease; acute glomerulonephritis; scleroderma; preeclampsia
- Endocrine: pheochromocytoma, Cushing's
- Sympathomimetics: cocaine, amphetamines, MAO inhibitors + foods rich in tyramine
- Cerebral injury: do *not* treat HTN in acute ischemic stroke unless Pt getting lysed, extreme BP (>220/120), Ao dissection, active ischemia or HF (*Stroke* 2003;34:1056)

Treatment (*Chest* 2007;131:1949)
- Tailor goals to clinical context (eg, more rapid lowering for Ao dissection)
- Emergency: ↓ MAP by ~25% in mins to 2 h w/ IV agents (may need arterial line for monitoring); goal DBP <110 w/in 2–6 h, as tolerated
- Urgency: ↓ BP to ≤160/100 in hrs using PO agents; goal normal BP in ~1–2 d
- Watch UOP, Cr, mental status: may indicate a lower BP is not tolerated

Drugs for Hypertensive Crises		
IV	Nitroprusside* 0.25–10 mcg/kg/min	Nitroglycerin 5–1000 mcg/min
	Labetalol 20–80 mg IVB q10min or 0.5–2 mg/min	Esmolol 0.5 mg/kg load → 0.05–0.2 mg/kg/min
	Fenoldopam 0.1–1.6 mcg/kg/min	Hydralazine 10–20 mg q20–30 min
	Nicardipine 5–15 mg/h	Clevidipine 1–16 mg/h
	Phentolamine 5–15 mg bolus q5–15min	Enalaprilat 1.25 mg
PO	Captopril 12.5–100 mg tid	Labetalol 200–800 mg tid
	Clonidine 0.2 mg load → 0.1 mg qh	Hydralazine 10–75 mg qid

*Metabolized to cyanide →Δ MS, lactic acidosis, death. Limit use of very high doses (8–10 mcg/kg/min) to <10 min. Monitor thiocyanate levels. Hydroxocobalamin or sodium thiosulfate infusion for treatment of cyanide toxicity.

Treatment Considerations for Specific Clinical Settings		
Clinical Setting	**Note**	**Treatment**
Acute stroke	BP ↓ must be balanced w/ risk of worsening ischemia	Consult stroke team
Aortic dissection (qv)	✓ BP in both arms and treat higher value	**βB first**, then add vasodilator (eg, nitroprusside) if needed
Acute pulm edema	Avoid ⊖ inotropes (eg, βB) if LV dysfxn, unless ischemia	Vasodilator (eg, NTG) and loop diuretic
Antihypertensive withdrawal	Suspect if abrupt d/c of symp. blocker (eg, clonidine)	Restart d/c'd drug or consider labetalol or nitroprusside
Sympathetic activity (pheo, auton dysfxn, cocaine, MAO + tyramine-containing foods)	**Avoid βB** as could → unopposed α in vasculature → vasoconstriction and further ↑ BP	Phentolamine (pheochromocytoma), nitroprusside

RENOVASCULAR DISEASE

Pathophysiology
- ↓ renal perfusion → activation of RAA system → vasoconstriction, ↑ aldo & vasopressin, ↑ sympathetic activity → volume retention & HTN → progressive renal dysfxn and CV risk
- Unilateral stenosis → HTN
- Bilateral (or unilat involving solitary functioning kidney) → HTN & progressive renal insuffic

Etiologies
- **Atherosclerosis** (~90%): usually involving ostial or prox segments. Often incidental finding as common in Pts w/ established athero (eg, CAD, PAD) but uncommon cause of HTN.
- **Fibromusclar dysplasia** (FMD, ~10%): nonathero medial fibroplasia usually mid/distal female-predominant (85-90%); mean age 52 y (Circ 2012;125:3182)
  characteristic "string of beads" appearance (or concentric smooth stenosis) on angio usually >1 territory involved (eg, carotid in ~65%), explaining sx of HA, dizziness, tinnitus
- **Other** (uncommon): vasculitis (Takayasu's, GCA, PAN or eosinophilic granulomatosis w/ polyangiitis) often w/ ↑ inflammatory markers, systemic s/s; scleroderma; local aneurysm or dissection; embolism; retroperitoneal fibrosis

Diagnosis
- Consider testing if any of the following *and* if finding would modify treatment:
  Clinical picture consistent w/ secondary HTN w/ no other compelling etiology
  Severe HTN (SBP ≥180 and/or DBP ≥120 mmHg) and/or flash pulm edema/CHF
  Progressive renal insufficiency w/ bland sediment, unilateral small kidney (≤9 cm), renal asymmetry >1.5 cm, or acute sustained Cr ↑ by ≥30% w/in 1 wk of starting ACEI/ARB

Testing for Renovascular Disease (Am Fam Physician 2009;80:273)			
Modality	**Se**	**Sp**	**Notes**
Duplex Doppler US	85%	92%	Pt habitus & operator dependent. May be preferred if renal dysfxn. Allows quantification of resistive index.*
CTA	88–96%	97%	Less sensitive (~30%) for distal disease such as FMD Contrast agent nephrotoxic
MRA	88–100%	>95%	Less sensitive (~30%) for distal disease such as FMD Risk of nephrogenic systemic fibrosis if mod-sev CKD
Angiography (DSA)	gold standard		Allows measurement of gradients Invasive, contrast agent nephrotoxic
Plasma Renin Activity (PRA)	50–80%	low	Not 1st line. Can ↑ Se by measuring 1 hr after capto administration
Captopril Renal Scan	75–100%	n/a	Not 1st line, but can determine hemodynamic signif of stenosis. Not reliable in bilateral RAS or poor renal fxn.

*Resistive index = [(peak syst vel – end diast vel) / peak syst vel].

- Monitoring: for athero, repeat imaging only necessary if Δ in clinical status that would lead to intervention; for FMD image q6–12mo to assess for progression

Treatment
- If due to atherosclerosis, risk factor modification: quit smoking, ↓ chol
- Antihypertensive Rx effective for most Pts: diuretic + ACEI/ARB (watch for ↑ Cr) or CCB
- Revascularization (typically percutaneous w/ stenting):
  Had considered if refractory HTN, recurrent flash pulm edema, worsening CKD
  However, clinical trials enrolling stable Pts w/ mod stenosis (50–70%) and HTN on ≥2 agents showed no benefit on # of BP meds, renal fxn or CV outcomes (NEJM 2000;342:1007; 2009;361:1953; 2014;370:13). Unknown if beneficial in more severe stenoses or in higher-risk Pts (eg, recent CHF, >3 meds).
  Resistive index >80 on U/S implies intrinsic renal damage and thus less likely to benefit from revasc, so may predict outcome after intervention (NEJM 2001;344:410). Operator dependent and some studies have not replicated findings, so not utilized broadly.
  Renal vein renin measurements, PRA, captopril renogram may provide supportive evidence as to hemodynamic significance of RAS, but limited utility due to low Se For FMD (usually more distal lesions): PTA ± bailout stenting
- Surgery (very rare): resection of pressor kidney
- Bilateral RAS: 20–46% of Pts w/ RAS. Associated w/ higher creatinine and worse CV outcomes. In addition to anti-HTN Rx, consider revasc if likely to benefit (failure of meds, recurrent pulmonary edema, progressive renal failure). Trials including Pts w/ bilateral RAS did not show benefit but included moderate stenoses.

Definitions
- **True** aneurysm (≥50% dilation of all 3 layers of aorta; <50% called ectasia) vs **false or pseudoaneurysm** (rupture contained by adventitia)
- **Location:** root (annuloaortic ectasia), thoracic aortic aneurysm (TAA), thoracoabdominal aortic aneurysm (TAAA), abdominal aortic aneurysm (AAA)
- **Type:** fusiform (circumferential dilation) vs saccular (localized dilation of aortic wall)

Epidemiology (Circ 2010;121:e266, 2011;124:2020 & 2013;127:e6; Nat Rev Cardiol 2011;8:92)
- In U.S., ~15,000 deaths/y from aortic ruptures; overall ~50,000 deaths/y from Ao disease
- **TAA:** 10/100,000 Pt-yrs, ♂:♀ 2:1; ~60% root/ascending; 40% descending
- **AAA:** ~4–8% prev in those >60 y (although may be ↓; Circ 2011;124:1118);
  4–6× more common in ♂ vs ♀; mostly infrarenal
- Arch & TAAA rarer

Pathophysiology (NEJM 2009;361:1114; Nat Med 2009;15:649)
- Medial degeneration and/or ↑ wall stress
  Medial degeneration = muscle apoptosis, elastin fiber weakening, mucoid infiltration
  Wall stress ∝ [(ΔP × r) / (wall thickness)], LaPlace's law
- **TAA:** most commonly medial degeneration; seen w/ connective tissue disorders & aortitis
- **AAA:** most commonly long-standing HTN + athero/inflammation → medial weakening

Risk factors
- Classic: **HTN, atherosclerosis, smoking, age, male sex**
- **Marfan syndrome** (mutations in fibrillin-1, *FBN-1*): cardinal features are Ao root aneurysm & ectopia lentis. Other suggestive signs include: tall stature; arachnodactyly w/ *thumb sign* (entire distal phalanx of adduct. thumb extends beyond ulnar border of palm) and/or *wrist sign* (tip of thumb covers 5th finger fingernail when wrapped around contralat wrist); pectus deformities; scoliosis; dural ectasia; spontaneous PTX; MVP.
- **Loeys-Dietz syndrome** (mutation in TGF-β receptors 1 or 2, *TGFBR1/2*): triad of arterial tortuosity & aneurysms, widely spaced eyes, bifid uvula or cleft palate. Also w/ velvety & hyperlucent skin and bluish sclera.
- Vascular **Ehlers-Danlos syndrome** (mutation in type III procollagen, *COL3A1*): easy bruising; thin, translucent skin w/ visible veins (but not excessively stretchable); acrogeria (aged appearance of hands & feet); flexible digits; uterine or intestinal rupture; distinctive facial features (protruding eyes, thin nose & lips, sunken cheeks, small chin)
- Other genetic disorders: **bicuspid AoV**; Turner syndrome (45X; short stature, ovarian failure, Ao coarctation); other familial aortopathies (mutations in smooth muscle myosin & actin genes including MYH11 and ACTA2)
- **Aortitis:** Takayasu's, GCA, spondyloarthritis, IgG4-related disease
- **Infection** (ie, mycotic aneurysm): salmonella, TB, syphilis

Screening (Circ 2010;121:e266 & 2011;124:2020; Annals 2014;161:281; JAMA 2015;313:1156)
- **TAA:** if bicuspid AoV or 1° relative w/: (a) TAA or bicuspid valve, (b) Marfan, Loeys-Dietz, Turner; known relevant genetic mutation (see above)
- **AAA:** ✓ for pulsatile abd mass; U/S ♂ >60 y w/ FHx of AAA & ♂ 65–75 y w/ prior tobacco

Diagnostic studies (Circ 2010;121:e266 & 2011;124:2020)
- **Contrast CT:** quick, noninvasive, high Se & Sp for all aortic aneurysms
- **TTE/TEE:** TTE most useful for root and proximal Ao; TEE can visualize other sites of TAA
- **MRI:** preferred over CT for aortic root imaging for TAA; also useful in AAA but time-consuming; noncontrast "black blood" MR to assess aortic wall
- **Abdominal U/S:** screening and surveillance test of choice for infrarenal AAA

Treatment principles (Circ 2006;113:e463; 2008;117:1883; 2010;121:1544 & e266)
- Goal is to prevent rupture (50% mortality prior to hospital) by modifying risk factors
- **Smoking cessation:** smoking associated w/ ↑ rate of expansion (Circ 2004;110:16)
- **Statin** (to achieve LDL-C <70 mg/dL): ↓ death and stroke & possibly ↓ rate of expansion (Eur J Vasc Endovasc Surg 2006;32:21)
- **BP control:** βB (↓ dP/dt) ↓ aneurysm growth (NEJM 1994;330:1335)
  ACEI a/w ↓ risk of rupture (Lancet 2006;368:659)
  ARB may ↓ rate of aortic root growth in Marfan (NEJM 2008;358:2787)
  βB and ARB similar ↓ rate of Ao root growth in children and young adults w/ Marfan (NEJM 2014;371:2061)

- Moderate cardiovascular exercise okay, but no burst activity/exercise requiring Valsalva maneuvers (eg, heavy lifting)
- **Indications for intervention** (surgery/endovascular repair)
  - Individualize based on FHx, body size, gender, anatomy, surgical risk
  - **TAA** (Circ 2010;121:1544 & e266)
    - symptoms
    - ascending Ao ≥5.5 cm (4–5 cm if Marfan, bicuspid AoV, Loeys-Dietz, vascular EDS, or other genetic/familial disorder)
    - descending >6 cm
    - ↑ >0.5 cm/y
    - aneurysm >4.5 cm and planned AoV surgery
  - **AAA** (NEJM 2002;346:1437 & 2014;371:2101)
    - symptoms
    - infrarenal ≥5.5 cm, but consider ≥5.0 cm in ♀
    - ↑ >0.5 cm/y; inflam/infxn

Surgery (Circ 2010;121:e266; EHJ 2014;25:2873)
- Ascending aorta
  - No root involvement: resection & replacement w/ Dacron tube graft
  - Root involvement: need to address AoV integrity; depending on AoV itself:
    - modified Bentall: Dacron Ao root + prosthetic AoV, reattach coronaries
    - valve-sparing: reimplant native AoV in Dacron Ao graft; reattach coronaries
- Arch: high-risk, complex surgery because of the arch branches; variety of combinations of partial/complete resection, stent graft & bypass of arch vessels
- Descending thoracic aorta: resection & grafting vs endovascular repair (qv)

Endovascular repair (EVAR) (NEJM 2008;358:494; Circ 2011;124:2020 & 2015;131:1291)
- Depends on favorable aortic anatomy
- TEVAR (thoracic EVAR) for descending TAA ≥5.5 cm may ↓ periop morbidity and possibly mortality (Circ 2010;121:2780; JACC 2010;55:986; J Thorac CV Surg 2010;140:1001 & 2012;144:604)
- AAA
  - Guidelines support open repair or EVAR for infrarenal AAA in good surg candidates
  - ↓ short-term mort., bleeding, LOS; but long-term graft complic. (3–4%/y; endoleak, need for reintervention, rupture) necessitate periodic surveillance, with no proven Δ in overall mortality in trials, except ? in those <70 y (NEJM 2010;362:1863, 1881 & 2012;367:1988)
  - In observational data, EVAR assoc w/ ↑ survival over 1st 3 y, after which survival similar. Rates of rupture over 8 y 5.4% w/ EVAR vs 1.4% w/ surgery (NEJM 2015;373:328)
  - In Pts unfit for surgery or high periop risks: ↓ aneurysm-related mortality but no Δ in overall mortality over medical Rx (NEJM 2010;362:1872). EVAR noninferior (? superior) to open repair in ruptured AAA w/ favorable anatomy (Ann Surg 2009;250:818).
- Pt selection for endovascular repair includes requirement to comply with long-term surveillance

Complications (Circ 2010;121:e266; Nat Rev Cardiol 2011;8:92)
- **Pain:** gnawing chest, back or abdominal pain; new or worse pain may signal rupture
- **Rupture:** risk ↑ w/ diameter, ♀, current smoking, HTN
  - **TAA:** ~2.5%/y if <6 cm vs 7%/y if >6 cm
  - **AAA:** ~1%/y if <5 cm vs 6.5%/y if 5–5.9 cm
  - rupture p/w severe constant pain and hemorrhagic shock; ~80% mortality at 24 h
- **Aortic insufficiency (TAA) and CHF**
- **Acute aortic syndromes** (qv)
- **Thromboembolic ischemic events** (eg, to CNS, viscera, extremities)
- **Compression of adjacent structures** (eg, SVC, trachea, esophagus, laryngeal nerve)

Follow-up (Circ 2010;121:1544 & e266; Nat Rev Cardiol 2011;8:92; JAMA 2013;309:806)
- Expansion rate ~0.1 cm/y for TAA, ~0.3–0.4 cm/y for AAA
- AAA: <4 cm q2–3 yrs; 4–5.4 cm q6–12 mos; more frequent if rate of expansion >0.5 cm in 6 mo
- TAA: 6 mo after dx to ensure stable, and if stable, then annually (Circ 2005;111:816)
- Screen for CAD, PAD and aneurysms elsewhere, espec popliteal. About 25% of Pts w/ TAA will also have AAA, and 25% of AAA Pts will have a TAA: consider pan-Ao imaging.
- Patients with endovascular repair require long-term surveillance for endoleak & to document stability of aneurysm

ACUTE AORTIC SYNDROMES

Definitions (Circ 2005;112:3802 & 2010;121:e266; Eur Heart J 2012;33:26)
- **Aortic dissection** (AoD): intimal tear → blood extravasates into Ao media (creates false lumen). Rate 3–16/100,000 Pt-yrs. False lumen acts as "wind sock," ↑ in size and compressing true lumen (patency of false lumen associated with outcome).
- **Intramural hematoma** (IMH): vasa vasorum rupture → medial hemorrhage that does not communicate with aortic lumen; 6% of aortic syndromes; clinically managed as AoD
- **Penetrating ulcer** (PAU): atherosclerotic plaque penetrates elastic lamina → medial hemorrhage. PAU in setting of IMH assoc. w/ similar outcomes as AoD. Outcomes for isolated PAU less well defined but considered AAS. Rx depends on clinical context.

Classification (proximal twice as common as distal)
- **Proximal:** involves ascending Ao, regardless of origin (= Stanford A, DeBakey I & II)
- **Distal:** involves descending Ao only, distal to L subclavian art. (= Stanford B, DeBakey III)
- **Other Considerations:** isolated to arch generally treated as proximal; distal with involvement of subclavian depends on overall clinical picture.

Risk factors
- **Classic** (in older Pts): **hypertension** (h/o HTN in >70% of dissections); **age** (60s–70s), **male sex** (~70% ♂); **smoking**
- **Genetic or acquired predisposition** (may present younger; see "Aortic Aneurysms"):
  Connective tissue disease/congenital anomaly: Marfan, Loeys-Dietz, vascular Ehlers-Danlos, bicuspid AoV, coarctation (eg, in Turner's), other familial aortopathies, PCKD
  Aortitis: Takayasu's, GCA, Behçet's, syphilis
  Pregnancy: typically 3rd trimester
- Other environmental factors:
  Trauma: blunt, deceleration injury
  Cardiovascular procedures: IABP, cardiac or aortic surgery, cardiac catheterization
  Acute ↑ BP: cocaine, Valsalva (eg, weightlifting)

Clinical Manifestations and Physical Exam* (JAMA 2000;283:897)		
Feature	**Proximal**	**Distal**
"Aortic" pain (abrupt, severe, tearing or ripping quality, *maximal at onset* [vs crescendo for ACS])	**94%** (chest, back)	**98%** (back, chest, abd)
Syncope (often due to tamponade)	13%	4%
HF (usually due to acute AI)	9%	3%
CVA	6%	2%
HTN	36%	70%
HoTN or shock (tamponade, AI, MI, rupture)	25%	4%
Pulse deficit (if involves carotid, subclavian, fem)	19%	9%
AI murmur	44%	12%

*S/S correlate w/ affected branch vessels & distal organs; may Δ as dissection progresses.

Initial evaluation (Circ 2010;121:e266)
- H&P, including bilateral BP and radial pulses for symmetry
  High-risk conditions: Marfan, CTD, FHx AoD, recent Ao manip., AoV dis., Ao aneurysm
  High-risk pain features: chest, back or abd pain described as [both (abrupt onset or severe intensity) and (ripping, tearing, sharp or stabbing) (absence ⊖ LR 0.3)]
  High-risk exam features:
    perfusion deficit [pulse deficit (⊕ LR 5.7), systolic BP differential (>20 mmHg), or focal neuro deficit + pain (⊕ LR >6)], or
    murmur of AI (new or not known to be old and in conjunction w/ pain), or
    hypotension or shock
- 12-lead ECG: often abnl but non-dx; may show STE if prox AoD involving coronary
- CXR: abnl in 60–90% [↑ mediast. (absence ⊖ LR 0.3), L pl effusion] but *cannot r/o AoD*
- *Obtain expedited Ao imaging if:* ≥2 high-risk features, 1 high-risk feature w/o clear alternative dx, or 0 features but unexplained HoTN or widened mediastinum on CXR

Diagnostic studies (Circ 2010;121:e266; JACC CV Img 2014;7:406)
- **CT:** quick, noninvasive, readily available, Se ≥93% & Sp 98%; however, if ⊖ & high clin. suspicion → additional studies (²/₃ w/ AoD have ≥2 studies; AJC 2002;89:1235)
- **MRI:** Se & Sp >98%, but time-consuming test & not readily available
- Axial studies (CT, MRI) should be gated to ECG to evaluate Ao root; if high index of suspicion, study should include entire aorta (chest, abd, & pelvis)

- **Echo**
  TTE: low Se (∴ not dx study) but can show effusion, AI, & dissection flap (if proximal)
  TEE: Se >95% prox, 80% for distal; can assess cors/peric/AI; "blind spot" behind trachea
- **Aortography**: Se ~90%, time-consuming, cannot detect IMH; can assess branch vessels
- **D-dimer**: Se/NPV ~97%; ? <500 ng/mL to r/o dissec (Circ 2009;119:2702) but not in Pts at high clinical risk (doi:10.1016/j.annemergmed.2015.02.013); does not r/o IMH

Initial medical treatment (Lancet 2008;372:55; Circ 2010;121:1544; JACC 2013;61:1661)
- ↓ dP/dt targeting HR <60 & central BP <120 (or lowest that preserves perfusion; r/o pseudohypotension, eg, arm BP ↓ due to subclavian dissection; use highest BP reading)
- **First** with IV βB (eg, esmolol, labetalol) to blunt reflex ↑ HR & inotropy that would occur in response to vasodilators; verap/dilt if βB contraindic.
- **Then** ↓ SBP with IV vasodilators (eg, nitroprusside)
- HTN control may require multiple agents (median of 4 in one study; J Hum Hypertens 2005;19:227). If unable to control readily: 1st evaluate for complication (eg, visceral ischemia); Rx pain w/ MSO₄; if no complication, then consider other drivers (eg, EtOH withdrawal).
- **If HoTN:** urgent surgical consultation, IVF to achieve euvolemia, pressors to keep MAP 70 mmHg; r/o complication (eg, tamponade, contained rupture, severe AI)

Treatment of proximal AoD (Circ 2010;121:1544; Lancet 2015;385:800)
- Acute: all cases should be considered for emergent surgery
  root replacement; valve sparing unless bicuspid or valve involvement
  acute stroke should not necessarily dissuade from surgery (mortality w/o surgery ~100%, Circ 2013;128:S175)
  prior AoV surgery postulated to be protective from complications, but most would operate
  need for preop coronary angio debatable as procedure nontrivial in setting of dissection and likelihood of performing concomitant CABG low
- Chronic: consider surgery if complicated by progression, AI or aneurysm

Treatment of distal AoD (Circ 2010;121:1544; JACC 2013;61:1661; Lancet 2015;385:800)
- Intervention warranted if complication (see below)
- Endovascular intervention (fenestrate flap to decompress false lumen, open occluded branch, stent entry tear) may be preferred over surgery due to possible ↓ mort. (JACC 2013;61:1661 & Circ 2015;131:1291)
- Stent graft for uncomplicated cases may ↓ risk of aorta-related complications and adverse remodeling (Circ Cardiovasc Interven 2013;6:407)

Complications (occur in ~20%; Circ 2003;108:II-312 & 2010;121:e266)
- Monitor all Pts w/ frequent assessment (sx, BP, UOP), pulse exam, labs (Cr, Hb, lactic acid), imaging (~7 d or sooner if sx or significant lab Δ)
- Uncontrolled BP despite intensive IV Rx or continued or ↑ pain may indicate complication
- **Progression:** propagation of dissection, ↑ aneurysm size, ↑ false lumen size
- **Rupture:** pericardial sac → tamponade (avoid pericardiocentesis unless PEA); blood in pleural space, mediast., retroperitoneum; ↑ in hematoma on imaging portends rupture
- **Malperfusion** (partial or complete obstruction of branch artery)
  can be static (avulsed/thrombosed) or dynamic (Δs in pressure in true vs false lumen)
  coronary → MI (usually RCA → IMI, since dissection often along outer Ao curvature)
  innominate/carotid → CVA, Horner
  intercostal/lumbar → spinal cord ischemia/paraplegia
  innominate/subclavian → upper extremity ischemia; iliac → lower extremity ischemia
  celiac/mesenteric → bowel ischemia (can be subtle w/ nonspecific GI sx, anorexia, pain)
  renal → acute renal failure or diguria/↑ Cr, refractory HTN
- **AI:** due to annular dilatation or disruption or displacement of leaflet by false lumen
- Mortality (Circ 2013;127:2031; JACC 2015;66:350)
  ~50% prior to hospital
  historically ~1%/h × 48 h for acute prox AoD who survive to hospital w/ 47% subseq mort at 30 d; more recent data w/ 22% in-hospital mortality
  13% at 30 d for acute distal overall but 25% if complications
  mortality similar for proximal and distal that survive to discharge: ~85% at 5 y

Long-term monitoring
- Major concern is progression to aneurysm or recurrent dissection
- Treat BP, risk factors aggressively
- **Serial imaging for all** (CT or MRI, latter may be preferred to lower cumulative radiation exposure) at 1, 3, and 6 mo, and then annually (18 mo, 30 mo, etc.)
- Pts treated endovascularly need close follow-up to monitor for complication (eg, endoleak)
- Partial thrombosis of false lumen associated with worse outcomes/mortality (NEJM 2007;357:349)
- In patients who present at young age or other indications of predisposing factor, consider genetic evaluation and screening of family members

PERIPHERAL ARTERY DISEASE (PAD)

Epidemiology and risk Factors
- Prev. ↑ w/ age: <1% if <40 y, ~15% if ≥70 y; risk factors incl. **smoking, DM**, HTN, chol
- More frequent in Pts w/ other symptomatic atherosclerotic disease (eg, coronary, carotid)
- Associated w/ ↑ risk of CV events (*JAMA* 2007;297:1197)
- If sx, 3-y risk of stroke ~3%, acute limb ischemia ~4%, periph revasc ~22% (*Circ* 2013;112:679)

Clinical Features
- **Asymptomatic** (~35%) or **atypical** sx (~40%): often undertreated in terms of risk factor modifying therapy (*Circ* 2011;124:17)
- **Claudication** (~25%): dull ache, often in calves
  precip by walking & relieved by stopping (vs spinal stenosis, qv)
  Leriche syndrome (aortoiliac occlusive disease): buttock & thigh claudication, ↓ or ∅ femoral pulses, & erectile dysfxn
- **Critical limb ischemia** (CLI, 1-2%): 1 or more of the following 3 manifestations
  rest pain: ↑ w/ elevation b/c ↓ perfusion
  ulcer: typically at pressure foci, often dry (in contrast, venous ulcers are more often at medial malleolus, wet, and with hemosiderin deposition)
  gangrene: more typically "dry" (ie, distal limb, dry shrunken and dark red, lack of pus) as a manifestation of ischemia due to impaired blood flow rather than "wet" (ie, infected, pus present, fetid smell), which may occur in the setting of infection or injury
  may be chronic (ie, sx >2-wk duration) vs acute limb ischemia, which is a *vascular emergency* (see below)
  a/w poor outcome: 45% amputation & 20% mortality at 6 mo (*J Vasc Surg* 2000;31:S1)
- Blue toe syndrome: most likely atheroembolic disease with occlusion of digital arteries

PAD Clinical Symptom Classification				
Rutherford		**Fontaine**		**Typical ABI***
Stage	**Definition**	**Stage**	**Definition**	
0	Asx	1	Asx	0.9–1.0
1	Mild claudication	2a	Sx at distance >650 ft	0.4–0.9
2	Mod claudication			
3	Severe claudication	2b	Sx at distance <650 ft	
4	Rest pain	3	Nocturnal or rest pain	<0.4
5	Ischemic ulceration not exceeding ulcer on digits of foot	4	Necrosis (death of tissue) and/or gangrene of limb	
6	Severe ischemic ulcers or frank gangrene			

*ABI is generally, but not absolutely correlated w/ clinical measures of lower extremity fxn & sx

Diagnosis
- Ddx includes
  nonvascular:
    neurogenic claudication (spinal stenosis): pain w/ standing, relieved by sitting, lying, or forward flexion; a/w neurologic abnl (weakness, sensory Δs, h/o deg. disc disease)
    musculoskeletal/arthritis: joint pain, morning stiffness, associated joint pathology or instability, crepitus or effusion
    Baker's cyst: posterior knee pain, knee stiffness, mass behind knee, discomfort w/ prolonged standing, impairment of bending
  non-athero vascular:
    venous claudication (uncommon): pain w/ walking in setting of proximal venous obstruction & no arterial obstruction
    dissection, embolism, aneurysm, or vasculitis
    popliteal artery entrapment (exercise-induced lower leg pain)
- Physical exam: ↓ peripheral pulses ± femoral bruits
  if severe: pallor of feet w/ elevation, dependent rubor, cyanosis
  other signs of chronic PAD: hair loss/shiny or cool skin, skin atrophy, nail hypertrophy

Testing
- **Ankle:brachial index (ABI):** nl 1–1.4; borderline 0.91–0.99; abnl ≤0.90; if >1.4, non-dx, likely due to calcified/noncompressible vessel
- **Toe:brachial index (TBI)** helpful if noncompressible (toe artery less likely to calcify); but ranges different than ABI (>0.7 nml, 0.5–0.7 mild, 0.35–0.5 mod, <0.35 mod–severe, severe if toe pressure <30 mmHg)

- **Segmental pressures** to determine level of disease (20 mmHg gradient between segments indicates stenosis)
- **Pulse volume recording (PVR)** done w/ segmental pressures: determine site and severity of disease. Abnormal waveform can indicate disease in noncompressible vessel, but pressures used over waveform if vessels are compressible.
- If ⊕ sx but nl ABI: **✓ exercise ABI** (some consider even in asx Pt w/ risk factors for PAD if will modify therapy)
- Treadmill study (or 6-min walk test) to quantify magnitude of functional limitation
- **Imaging** (Duplex arterial U/S; CTA w/ distal run-off; MRA or angio) if dx in question or considering intervention. Some do routine Duplex U/S to monitor graft/stent patency.

Medical treatment (JACC 2013;61:1555; JAMA 2013;309:453; Circ Res 2015;116:1579)
- **Treat risk factors:** smoking cessation, high-intensity statin, control HTN & DM, smoking cessation (JACC 2010;56:2105). βB OK if indicated for another reason (eg, CAD, AF).
- **Antiplatelet Rx:** benefit shown primarily for ↓ CV risk (BMJ 2002;324;71)
   If asx: benefit of antiplt Rx unclear espec if ABI only borderline (JAMA 2010;303;9)
   If sx: ASA or clopidogrel
      ASA: 23% ↓ risk of major CV events seen in meta-analysis of older studies (mostly ASA but also other antiplatelet Rx) (BMJ 2002;324;71)
      Clopidogrel: superior to ASA, but single, older study (Lancet 1996;348:1333)
      ASA+clopi may be better than ASA alone, but only posthoc study (EHJ 2009;30:1992)
      Vorapaxar (PAR-1 antag.) further ↓ risk on top of ASA or clopidogrel (Circ 2013;112:679)
- Anticoagulation w/ warfarin not beneficial (NEJM 2007;357:217)
- **ACEI/ARB** to ↓ CV risk (NEJM 2000;342:145)
- **Improve claudication**
   Supervised exercise: sx-limited, ≥3×/wk, ≥30–45 min/session, ↑ as tolerated; beneficial including ↑ walking time 50–200% (Cochrane 2014;7:CD990); structured exercise more effective than home-based, but home-based still effective (eg, JAMA 2013;310:57)
   ACEI & statins may ↓ sx (Circ 2003;108:1481)
   Cilostazol (nb, interacts w/ diltiazem & omeprazole; may cause headache or diarrhea; do not use in Pts w/ CHF); pentoxifylline likely less effective
- **Limb preservation:** foot exams for ulcers/wounds, revasc (qv), vorapaxar (PAR-1 antag) ↓ acute limb ischemia (Circ 2013;112:679), statin use assoc. w/ ↓ amput (EHJ 2014;35:2864)

Revascularization
- Consider if limiting sx despite exercise/medical Rx or if CLI; also consider as 1st-line Rx for isolated aortoiliac disease given high rate of long-term patency (Circ 2013;128:2704)
- **Endovascular** (angioplasty or stenting) usually favored over **surgical** (bypass or endarterectomy), but depends on lesion complexity & location (aortoiliac or "inflow" vs infrainguinal or "outflow") and Pt comorbidities
- Decision for stent vs angioplasty alone depends on lesion length & complexity, location (eg, over joints) (J Vasc Surg 2007;33:S1)
- Angioplasty w/ paclitaxel-coated balloon associated with ↑ primary patency vs regular balloon for femoropopliteal disease (NEJM 2015;373:145)
- Durability of endovascular revascularization depends in part on location, with greater long-term patency for iliac vs femoral interventions (JACC 2006;47:e1)
- Dual antiplatelet (DAPT, ASA + clopidogrel) commonly prescribed after endovascular intervention for 1–3 mo, but no prospective data. DAPT after bypass surgery not beneficial overall but possibly in subgroup w/ prosthetic grafts (J Vasc Surg 2010;52:825).
- Anticoagulation with warfarin does not improve patency (NEJM 2007;357:217), but may be indicated in subgroups with high thrombotic risk
- Stents not ferromagnetic, so MRI safe, but both MRI & CT may have artifact. Duplex U/S useful to assess stent patency and is used by some for serial routine monitoring of stent or graft patency, even in asx Pts.
- If coronary angiography needed, avoid access through CFA stent or femoral bypass

Acute limb ischemia (ALI)
- Sudden decrement in limb perfusion that threatens viability;
   viable (no imminent threat of tissue loss): audible art. Doppler signals, sensory & motor OK
   threatened (salvage requires prompt Rx): loss of arterial Doppler signal, sensory or motor
- Etiologies: embolism > acute thrombosis (eg, athero, APLA, HITT), trauma to artery
- Clinical manifestations (**6 Ps**): pain (distal to proximal, ↑ in severity), poikilothermia, pallor, pulselessness, paresthesias, paralysis
- Testing: thorough pulse & neuro exam; arterial Doppler; angiography, either CT w/ bilateral run-off through feet or arteriography
- Urgent consultation w/ vascular medicine and/or vascular surgery
- Treatment: immediate anticoagulation ± intra-arterial lytic; angioplasty or surgery

EXTRACRANIAL DISEASE

Pathobiology

- Involving portions of carotid or vertebral arteries outside skull. Most commonly at carotid bifurcation but may involve common (CCA), internal (ICA), or external carotid (ECA).
- Most common etiology is athero; others include FMD, vasculitis, dissection, & radiation
- Associated w/ ↑ risk of systemic CV events including ipsilateral TIA/stroke
- Progressive narrowing, thrombosis or unstable plaque in CCA or ICA → embolization and/or ↓ distal perfusion → ischemia → TIA/stroke
- Asx *chronically occluded* vessel associated w/ low risk, as no embolization and Circle of Willis provides collateral flow

Diagnosis (Circ 2011;124:354)

- Stenosis defined as % lumen diameter at most severe stenosis relative to either ICA, probable lumen diameter at site of stenosis, or proximal common carotid (*J Neuroimaging* 1994;4:222). Significant stenosis is >50%.
- Carotid bruit suggestive but not sensitive
- **Duplex U/S:** Se >80%, Sp ~85%; 1st-line test
  Peak systolic velocity (PSV) for severity
  ↑ end diastolic velocity (EDV), spectral broadening, carotid index (ratio of PSV in ICA vs CCA) and echolucent plaque each associated w/ ↑ risk
  PSV >200 cm/s + EDV >140 cm/s + carotid index >4.5 has Se 96% for significant stenosis (*Stroke* 1996;27:1965; *Mayo Clin Proc* 2000;75:1133)
- Transcranial Doppler (TCD) as adjunct to U/S may show severe stenosis, evidence of occlusion (collateral flow), or microemboli by high-intensity signal transients (HITS)
- If significant but nonsevere stenosis, repeat study at 6 mo to determine if stable and then annually thereafter
- If stenosis appears severe (≥70%) or requires further characterization, then either CT angio (Se ~90%, Sp ≥95%) or MRA (Se ~95%, Sp ≥95%). Caution with contrast & risk of either renal dysfxn (CTA) or nephrogenic systemic fibrosis (MRA).
- Angiography gold standard but invasive and assoc w/ risk of stroke

Asx carotid stenosis (Curr Treat Opt CV Med 2013;252:63; Expert Rev CV Ther 2014;12:437)

- Cause of <15% of strokes and risk <1% annually in Pts on standard med Rx (see below)
- General management
  lifestyle intervention (smoking cessation, diet modification, exercise)
  antiplatelet therapy: ASA 75–325 mg/d or clopidogrel 75 mg/d if ASA allergic (*Circ* 2011;124:354)
  high-intensity statin (see "Lipids") and **BP control** (see "HTN")
- **Revascularization** (see options below) for selected Pts w/ ≥70% stenosis
  older trials have shown ↓ stroke risk vs med Rx alone, but not compared to modern med Rx (*NEJM* 1993;328:221; *JAMA* 1995;273:1421; *Lancet* 2004;363:1491)
  due to low rate of associated stroke, absolute risk reduction likely small and benefit of intervention debated
  consider Pt preference, risk of procedure, overall life expectancy (eg, ≥5 y), gender (benefit less certain in women), lesion characteristics of ↑ stroke risk (eg, echolucent plaque, TCD evidence of microemboli)

Symptomatic carotid stenosis (NEJM 2013;369:12)

- Symptomatic stenosis indicative of severe/unstable plaque and associated w/ ↑ risk of stroke. ∴ determination of sx important regarding treatment plan.
- Defined as recent (<6 mo) focal neurologic sx, sudden in onset, referable to carotid distribution. May include TIA or minor stroke [incl amaurosis fugax (transient monocular blindness)]. Vertigo & syncope unlikely related and generally not considered sx.
- For acute treatment for stroke, see "Stroke"
- All Pts w/ sx stenosis should receive med Rx as above
- Revascularization (*NEJM* 1991;325:445; *Lancet* 2004;363:915)
  recommended for 70-99% stenosis, generally w/in 2 wk unless severe comorbidity w/ limited lifespan, severe ipsilateral stroke w/ persistent deficit, occluded carotid, or high operative risk (≥6%)
  consider for 50-69% stenosis, depending on Pt-specific factors
  not indicated if <50% stenosis

Revascularization options

- **Carotid endarterectomy** (CEA): gold standard. Risk of procedural stroke or death <3% for asymptomatic disease and <6% for sx disease in experienced centers.
- Carotid artery stenting (CAS; *JACC* 2014;64:722): compared w/ CEA, periprocedural risk of stroke ↑ (espec in elderly) & MI ↓ (although many asx), subsequent rates of stroke similar (*NEJM* 2010;363:11; *Lancet* 2010;376:1062). Consider if not surgical candidate (anatomy or comorbidities). Generally requires DAPT (ASA + clopidogrel) for 30 d.

INTRACRANIAL DISEASE

- Cerebral and basilar arteries and distal branches thereof
- Most common etiology is athero & assoc w/ traditional athero risk factors (*Circ* 2014;1407:14); others include: dissection, FMD, vasoconstriction, vasculitis, moyamoya
- Estimated to cause 5–10% of ischemic strokes and more prevalent among blacks, Hispanics and Asians (*Stroke* 1995;26:14)
- Diagnosis: MRA, CTA, or TCD vs angio (see above); duplex U/S not useful
- Medical treatment similar as in extracranial; however, consider ASA+clopidogrel for sx disease for 90 d (*NEJM* 2011;365:993)
- Stenting and intracranial bypass not shown to be beneficial and not routinely recommended (*NEJM* 2011;365:993; *JAMA* 2015;313:1240)

PHARMACOLOGIC SECONDARY STROKE PREVENTION

Antiplatelet therapy (*NEJM* 2012;366:1914)

- In general monotherapy preferred to multiagent therapy for long-term prevention due to ↑ ICH risk w/ multiagent therapy
- **ASA:** ↓ death & repeat stroke; equal to warfarin in nonembolic stroke (*NEJM* 2001;345:1444)
- **Clopidogrel:** marginally superior to ASA, slightly ↑ ICH (*Lancet* 1996;348:1329)
- **Multiagent antiplatelet therapy:**
  ASA + clopi: not more effective than ASA alone and ↑ bleeding & ICH (*Lancet* 2004;364:331; *NEJM* 2012;367:817). In minor stroke/TIA, ASA + clopi × 21 d → clopi monoRx vs ASA monoRx resulted in ↓ stroke w/o ↑ ICH (*NEJM* 2013;369:11).
  ASA + dipyridamole: superior to ASA (*Lancet* 2006;367:1665), but ↑ ICH and poor compliance
  Addition of vorapaxar to ASA or ASA+clopi ↓ first stroke in Pts w/ athero, but contra-indicated in patients w/ prior stroke due to ICH risk (*NEJM* 2012;366:1404; *Stroke* 2013;691:8)

Anticoagulation

- Not routinely indicated. Anticoag if cardiac/paradoxical emboli (except bacterial endocarditis) or hypercoag state. See "AF" and "VTE" for details.
- **Hold off on anticoag** in large strokes for ~2–4 wk given risk of hemorrhagic conversion.

Risk factor management

- BP (see "HTN"). long-term SBP target 120–139 mmHg (*JAMA* 2011;306:2137)
- LDL: high-intensity statin therapy (*Circ* 2014;129(Suppl 2).S1)

OTHER CEREBROVASCULAR DISEASES

Cervical artery dissection

- May involve intracranial or extracranial arteries. Manifests as luminal stenosis, thrombo-embolism or aneurysm. ~20% of ischemic strokes in young Pts (primarily embolic).
- Etiologies: trauma, physical activity, ? neck manip.; can be spontaneous (if assoc cond.)
- FMD most common assoc. condition (seen in 15–20%). Others infrequent: vascular EDS, Marfan, osteogenesis imperfect, homocystinuria, PKD, α_1-AT.
- Most (>60%) report HA or neck pain, Horner's in ~25%, tinnitus, rarely eye pain
- Imaging may show "crescent sign" of hematoma, string sign, tapering stenosis, flap or dissected aneurysm. Duplex U/S can be initial screen but lower Se (68–95%) and limited utility at skull base. CTA & MRA w/ similar Se & Sp; angio if inconclusive noninvasive imaging.
- Treatment: if stroke, see "Stroke." In general, thrombolysis should not be withheld if indicated. If SAH, manage accordingly.
- Antithrombotic therapy: either anticoagulation (AC) or antiplatelet Rx may be considered for extracranial dissection; however, large meta-analysis showed no benefit of AC over antiplatelet Rx (*Neurology* 2012;79:686). If AC chosen, typically for 3–6 mo, then Δ to antiplatelet. Intracranial dissection treated with antiplatelet monotherapy and not AC.
- Endovascular therapy or surgery considered for selected Pts, particularly if recurrent ischemia; however, no trials to demonstrate benefit.

Patent foramen ovale (PFO; in ~27% of population) *(NEJM 2005;353:2361)*

- ↑ stroke risk: ≥4-mm separation, R → L shunting at rest, ↑ septal mobility, atrial septal aneurysm
- If PFO & stroke/TIA: no benefit of warfarin over ASA *(Circ 2002;105:2625)*, but consider it at high risk for or has DVT/PE. No sig benefit shown for PFO closure so far, albeit studies small & w/ favorable trends *(NEJM 2012;366:991; 2013:1083 & 1092).*

Intracranial aneurysm *(Stroke 2015;46:2368)*

- Prevalence of saccular aneurysms 3.2%, w/ equal sex ratio *(Lancet Neurol 2011;10:626)*; 20–30% having >1 aneurysm
- Associated with family hx, hereditary syndromes (eg, EDS, polycystic kidney), smoking, HTN, aortic coarctation, ? estrogen deficiency (female preponderance after menopause) *(Stroke 2001;32:606)*
- Clinical presentations: most commonly incidental finding on brain imaging
    may be found in those presenting with SAH, which typically presents as "worst headache of my life," ± syncope, nausea, vomiting, meningismus *(Neurology 1986;36:1445)*
    rarely unruptured aneurysms become symptomatic (eg, headache, visual change, cranial neuropathy, facial pain)
- Diagnosis: CTA or MRA
- Instruct Pt to avoid smoking, heavy EtOH use, illicit drugs, straining/Valsalva
- Treatment requires consideration of size, location, Pt age and comorbidities. In general:
    if sx or SAH → repair
    if no sx/SAH and ≥7–10 mm, consider repair
    if <7 mm observe (CTA or MRA q6mo and every 2–3 y once showing no Δ)
    endovascular coiling ↓ periprocedural morbidity & mortality vs surgical clipping, but ↑ risk of recurrence

Extracranial aneurysm

- Rare (<1% of arterial aneurysms) *(Surgery 1983;93:319)*
- True aneurysm may be associated with athero, trauma, dissection (qv), infection, vasculitis or radiation. Male:female predominance (2:1).
- Infected pseudoaneurysm may occur at site of prior carotid intervention.
- Clinical presentation: TIA/stroke; less likely mass effect or rupture
- Diagnosis: see approach for carotid disease above
- Instruct Pt to avoid smoking, heavy EtOH use, illicit drugs, straining/Valsalva
- Treatment: sx disease should be repaired; consider repair if asx and >2 cm, w/ thrombus, or ≤2 cm but ↑'ing. Surgical and endovascular options depending on anatomy & Pt risk.

Cerebral venous thrombosis (CVT) *(Circ 2012;125:1709)*

- Uncommon (<2/100,000/yr); female predominance (3× more common)
- >85% w/ risk factor including: hypercoagulable state, OCP, pregnancy, malignancy, infection, prior trauma, vasculitis, other inflammatory states (eg, IBD), hematologic disorders, nephrotic syndrome
- Clinical presentation variable and includes HA (~90%), seizure, focal deficits, encephalopathy, sx of isolated intracranial hypertension (HA ± vomiting, papilledema, visual problems) may occur if hemorrhage or edema
- Diagnose w/ MR venography or CT venography (traditional head CT normal in ~30% of CVT). D-dimer may be elevated but does not reliably exclude.
- Acute treatment
    treat elevated ICP
    consider antiseizure Rx if seizure on presentation or otherwise high risk
    anticoagulation (UFH or LMWH; see VTE for dosing) if no contraindication (nb, presence of ICH not absolute contraindication)
    consider endovascular venous recanalization with direct thrombolysis if progressive neurologic worsening despite anticoagulation
- Chronic treatment
    anticoagulation w/ VKA w/ INR 2–3 for 3–6 mo if provoked or 6–12 if unprovoked
    consider indefinite duration if recurrent, complicated by DVT or PE, or severe thrombophilia
    if occurred in setting of OCP, change to nonestrogen-based contraception
- Monitoring: imaging at 3–6 mo after dx to assess for recanalization

VENOUS THROMBOEMBOLISM (VTE)

Definitions
- Superficial thrombophlebitis: pain, tenderness, erythema along superficial vein
- Deep venous thrombosis (DVT)
  - Proximal: thrombosis of iliac, femoral, or popliteal veins (nb, "superficial" femoral vein part of deep venous system)
  - Distal: calf veins below knee; lower risk of PE/death than prox (Thromb Haem 2009;102:493)
- Pulmonary embolism (PE): thrombosis originating in venous system and embolizing to pulmonary arterial circulation; 1 case/1000 person y; 250,000/y (Archives 2003;163:1711)

Risk factors
- Virchow's triad for thrombogenesis
  - **stasis:** bed rest, inactivity, CHF, CVA w/in 3 mo, air travel >6 h (NEJM 2001;345:779)
  - **injury to endothelium:** trauma, surgery, prior DVT, inflammation, central catheter
  - **thrombophilia:** APC resistance, protein C or S deficiency, APS, prothrombin gene mutation, ↑ factor VIII, hyperhomocysteinemia, HIT, OCP, HRT, tamoxifen, raloxifene
- Malignancy (12% of "idiopathic" DVT/PE)
- History of thrombosis (greater risk of recurrent VTE than genetic thrombophilia)
- Obesity, smoking, acute infection, postpartum (JAMA 1997;277:642; Circ 2012;125:2092)
- Statin therapy ↓ risk (NEJM 2009;360:1851)

Thromboprophylaxis (Chest 2012;141:e195S, 227S, 278S)	
Patient & situation	**Prophylaxis**
Low-risk med; same-day surg & <40 y	Early, aggressive ambulation
Minor surgery in mobile Pt	Mechanical Ppx
High-risk medical (eg, immobilized, h/o VTE, thrombophilia or cancer) Most surgery Pts	**UFH** 5000 U SC bid or tid, or **LMWH**, or fonda (if HIT ⊕), or mech Ppx (espec if high bleed risk)
High-risk surg (eg, trauma, recent stroke or spinal cord injury, h/o VTE or thrombophilia)	**[LMWH or UFH SC] + mech Ppx**
Orthopedic surgery	**LMWH** [or fonda, direct oral anticoag (qv) or warfarin (INR 2–3)] + mech Ppx. Start before or shortly after (<12 h) surgery & cont. up to **35 d** (hip) or **10–14 d** (knee). LMWH or fonda favored over UFH or VKA. Direct oral anticoagulants overall appear favorable vs LMWH.

For enoxaparin, 30 mg bid for highest risk or 40 mg qd for moderate risk or spinal/epidural anesth. Dose adjust: qd in CrCl <30 mL/min, ↑ 30% if BMI >40 (Ann Pharmacother 2009;43:1064).

- **Direct oral anticoagulants vs LMWH** (Annals 2012;156:710)
  - Dabigatran (approved in Europe & Canada); 110 mg 1–4 h after surgery & hemostasis or 220 mg if not initiated on day of surgery; 220 mg qd maintenance) noninferior to LMWH after hip and knee surgery (Lancet 2007;370:949)
  - Rivaroxaban (10 mg qd 6–10 h postop) ↓VTE by ≈25–50% vs enox 40 mg qd, with ≈ bleeding after hip or knee replacement (NEJM 2008;358:2765 & 2776; Lancet 2009;373:1673)
  - Apixaban (2.5 mg bid 12–24 h postop) ↓VTE by ≈50% vs enox 40 mg qd, with ≈ bleeding after hip replacement (NEJM 2010;363:2487)
  - Edoxaban (30 mg qd 6-24 h after surgery) ↓VTE vs enox 20 mg qd, but no comparison to standard dose enox (Thromb Res 2014;134:1198)
- Evolving role for Ppx in ambulatory cancer Pts w/ low bleeding risk and additional VTE risk factors (NEJM 2012;366:601). Khorana score (cancer site, plt & WBC counts, Hb, BMI) risk predictor (Blood 2008;111:4902). Semuloparin (ultra LMWH) ↓VTE by ≈2/3 w/o ↑ major bleeding in Pts w/ met. or locally adv. cancer receiving chemo (NEJM 2012;366:601).

Clinical manifestations—DVT
- Calf pain, swelling (>3 cm c/w unaffected side), venous distention, erythema, warmth, tenderness, palpable cord, ⊕ Homan's sign (calf pain on dorsiflexion, seen in <5%)
- *Phlegmasia cerulea dolens:* massive proximal DVT → stagnant blood → edema, *cyanosis,* pain, compartment syndrome → can lead to limb loss or death
- 50% of Pts w/ sx DVT have asx PE
- Palpable tender superficial veins c/w superficial thrombophlebitis rather than DVT
- Popliteal (Baker's) cyst: related to knee pathology, may result in calf pain & may lead to DVT due to compression of popliteal vein

"Simplified Wells" Pretest Probability Scoring of DVT (JAMA 2006;295:199)	
Clinical variable	**Point score**
• Active cancer (Rx ongoing or w/in 6 mo or palliative)	1
• Paralysis, paresis, or recent immobilization of lower extremities	1
• Recently bedridden for ≥3 d or major surgery w/in 12 wk	1
• Localized tenderness along distribution of deep venous system	1
• Entire leg swelling	1
• Calf ≥3 cm larger than asx calf (at 10 cm below tibial tuberosity)	1
• Pitting edema confined to sx leg	1
• Collateral superficial veins (nonvaricose)	1
• Previous DVT	1
• Alternative dx at least as likely as DVT	−2

Pretest Probability Assessment		
Score ≤0	Score 1 or 2	Score ≥3
Low probability (5%)	Moderate probability (17%)	High probability (53%)

• For UE DVT, +1 point each for venous cath, local pain, & unilateral edema, −1 if alternative dx. ≤1 = unlikely; ≥2 = likely. U/S if likely or if unlikely but abnl D-dimer (Annals 2014;160:451).

Diagnostic studies—DVT
• D-dimer: <500 helps r/o; ? use 1000 as threshold if low risk (Annals 2013;158:93)
• Compression U/S >95% Se & Sp for sx DVT (lower for asx DVT); survey whole leg rather than just proximal if ≥mod prob (JAMA 2010;303:438); venography rarely used

Figure 1-5 Approach to suspected DVT (Chest 2012;141:e351S)

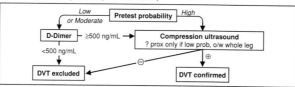

Clinical manifestations—PE
• Dyspnea (73%), pleuritic chest pain (66%), cough (37%), hemoptysis (13%)
• ↑ RR (>70%), crackles (51%), ↑ HR (30%), fever, cyanosis, pleural friction rub, loud P_2
• *Massive:* syncope, HoTN, PEA; ↑ JVP, R-sided S_3, Graham Steell (PR) murmur

Simplified Wells Pretest Probability Scoring for PE (Annals 2011;154:709)	
• Prior PE or DVT	• Clinical signs of DVT
• Active cancer	• HR >100 bpm
• Immobilization (bed rest ≥3 d) or surgery w/in 4 wk	• Hemoptysis
• Alternative dx less likely than PE	

Dichotomized Wells Probability Assessment	
≤1 Variable = "Unlikely" (13% probability)	> 1 Variable = "Likely" (39% probability)

Diagnostic studies—PE (NEJM 2010;363:266)
• CXR (limited Se & Sp): 12% nl, atelectasis, effusion, ↑ hemidiaphragm, Hampton hump (wedge-shaped density abutting pleura); Westermark sign (avascularity distal to PE)
• ECG (limited Se & Sp): sinus tachycardia, AF; signs of RV strain → RAD, P pulmonale, RBBB, $S_I Q_{III} T_{III}$ & TWI V_1–V_4 (McGinn-White pattern; Chest 1997;111:537)
• ABG: hypoxemia, hypocapnia, respiratory alkalosis, ↑ A-a gradient (Chest 1996;109:78), 18% w/ room air P_aO_2 85–105 mmHg, 6% w/ nl A-a gradient (Chest 1991;100:598)
• D-dimer (JAMA 2015;313:1668): high Se, poor Sp (~25%); ⊖ ELISA has >99% NPV ∴ use to r/o PE if "unlikely" pretest prob. (JAMA 2006;295:172) consider age-specific cutpoint: 500 if <50 y, 10× age if ≥50 y (JAMA 2014;311:1117)
• Echocardiography: useful for risk stratification (RV dysfxn), but not dx (Se <50%)
• V/Q scan: high Se (~98%), low Sp (~10%). Sp improves to 97% for high prob VQ. Use if pretest prob of PE high and CT not available or contraindicated. Can also exclude PE if low pretest prob, low prob VQ, but 4% false ⊖ (JAMA 1990;263:2753).
• CT angiography (CTA; see Radiology inserts; JAMA 2015;314:74): Se ~90% & Sp ~95% w/ MDCT (NEJM 2006;354:2317); PPV & NPV >95% if imaging concordant w/ clinical suspicion, ≤80% if discordant (∴ need to consider both); CT may also provide other dx
• Lower extremity compression U/S shows DVT in ~9%, sparing CTA, but when added to CTA, does not Δ outcomes (Lancet 2008;371:1343)

- Pulmonary angio: ? gold standard (morbidity 5%, mortality <0.5%), infrequently performed
- MR angiography: Se 84% (segmental) to 100% (lobar) (*Lancet* 2002;359:1643); if add MR venography, Se 92%, Sp 96% (*Annals* 2010;152:434)

Figure 1-6 Approach to suspected PE using CTA

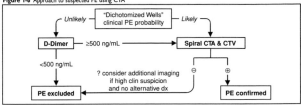

Based on data from *NEJM* 2005;352:1760 & 2006;354:22; *JAMA* 2005;293:2012 & 2006;295:172

Workup for idiopathic VTE
- **Thrombophilia workup:** ✓ if ⊕ FH, may be helpful but consider timing as thrombus, heparin and warfarin Δ results. May not be helpful for Pt if will not change management (eg, plan for long-term anticoagulation regardless), although could be of use to relatives (*JAMA* 2005;293:2352; *Blood* 2008;112:4432; *Am J Med* 2008;121:458).
- **Malignancy workup:** 12% Pts w/ "idiopathic" DVT/PE will have malignancy; age-appropriate screening adequate; avoid extensive w/u (*NEJM* 1998;338:1169 & 2015;373:697)

Risk stratification for Pts with PE
- **Clinical:** hypotension and/or tachycardia (~30% mortality), hypoxemia
- **CTA:** RV / LV dimension ratio >0.9 (*Circ* 2004;110:3276)
- **Biomarkers:** ↑ troponin & ↑ BNP a/w ↑ mortality; w/ ⊖ Tn, decomp extremely unlikely (*Circ* 2002;106:1263 & 2003;107:1576; *Chest* 2015;147:685)
- **Echocardiogram:** RV dysfxn (even if normal troponin) (*Chest* 2013;144:1539)
- **Simplified PE Severity Index:** 0 RFs → 1.1% mort.; ≥1 → 8.9% mort (*Archives* 2010;170:1383) RFs: age >80 y; h/o cancer; h/o HF or lung disease; HR ≥110; SBP <100; S_aO_2 <90%

Whom to treat (*Lancet* 2012;379;1835; *Chest* 2012;141:e419S)
- **Superficial venous thrombosis:** elevate extremity, warm compresses, compression stockings, NSAIDs for sx. Anticoag if high risk for DVT (eg, ≥5 cm, proximity to deep vein ≤5 cm, other risk factors) for 4 wk as ~10% have VTE w/in 3 mo (*Annals* 2010;152:218).
- **LE DVT:** proximal → anticoag. If distal: anticoag if severe sx, o/w consider serial imaging over 2 wk and anticoag if extends (although if bleeding risk low, many would anticoag).
- **UE DVT:** anticoagulate (same guidelines as LE; *NEJM* 2011;364:861). If catheter-associated, need not remove if catheter functional and ongoing need for catheter.
- **PE:** anticoagulate

Anticoagulation options (*Chest* 2012;141:e419S; *JAMA* 2014;311:717)
- Initiate immediately if high clinical suspicion or intermed but dx test results delayed for ≥4 h
- Either (a) initial parenteral anticoag → long-term oral anticoagulant (eg, warfarin or Xa inhibitor) or (b) solely with an oral Xa inhibitor
- **LMWH** (eg, enoxaparin 1 mg/kg SC bid or dalteparin 200 IU/kg SC qd)
  Preferred over UFH (espec in cancer) except: renal failure (CrCl <25), ? extreme obesity, hemodynamic instability or bleed risk (*Cochrane* 2004;CD001100)
  No need to monitor anti-factor Xa unless concern re: dosing (eg, renal insuffic.)
  Attractive option as outPt bridge to long-term oral anticoagulation
  If cancer, LMWH ↓ recur. & mort. c/w UFH & warfarin (*NEJM* 2003;349:146; *Lancet Oncol* 2008;9:577; *JAMA* 2015;314:677); ✓ head CT for brain mets if melanoma, renal, thyroid, chorioCA
- **Fondaparinux:** 5–10 mg SC qd (*NEJM* 2003;349:1695); use if HIT ⊕; avoid if renal failure
- DVT & low-risk PE can be treated completely as outPt (*Lancet* 2011;378:41)
- **IV UFH:** 80 U/kg bolus → 18 U/kg/h → titrate to PTT 1.5–2.3 × cntl (eg, 60–85 sec); preferred option when contemplating thrombolysis or catheter-based Rx (qv)
- IV Direct thrombin inhibitors (eg, argatroban, lepirudin) used in HIT ⊕ Pts
- **Warfarin** (goal INR 2–3): start same day as parenteral anticoag unless instability and ? need for lytic, catheter-based Rx or surgery; overlap ≥5 d w/ parenteral anticoag & until INR ≥2 × ≥24 h
- **Oral Xa inhibitor:** effect wears off w/in 24 h, but not easily immediately reversed
  Can give as sole anticoag (nb, dosing differs higher than for AF): **rivaroxaban** (15 mg bid for 1st 3 wk → 20 mg/d) as good/better than LMWH → warfarin in preventing recurrent VTE, ↓ bleeding (*NEJM* 2010;363:2499 & 2012;366:1287); **apixaban** (10 mg bid × 7 d → 5 bid) ≈ LMWH → warfarin in preventing recurrent VTE, ↓ bleeding (*NEJM* 2013;369:799)

*Can initiate after ≥5 d of parenteral anticoag (1st dose when d/c IV UFH or w/in 2 h before when next LMWH dose would have been due): both **dabigatran** (150 mg bid) & **edoxaban** (60 mg qd) ≈ warfarin but w/ ↓ bleeding (NEJM 2009;361:2342 & 2013;369:1406)*

Systemic thrombolysis (Chest 2012;141:e419S)
- Typically TPA 100 mg over 2 h or wt-adjusted TNK bolus
- Indications & efficacy below; risk of ICH ~1.5%, ↑ w/ age; see contraindications in "ACS"
- **Massive PE** (hemodynamic compromise): ↓ death and recurrent PE each by ~50% (Circ 2004;110:744; JAMA 2014;311:2414; EHJ 2015;36:605) & lower PVR long term (JACC 1990;15:65)
- **Submassive PE** (hemodyn. stable but RV dysfxn on echo or enlargement on CTA, or ? marked dyspnea or severe hypoxemia): ↓ death & ↑ bleeding; may consider if low bleed risk (see lytic contra-indic.; EHJ 2015;36:605). Benefit/risk may be more favorable if <75 y (NEJM 2014;370:1402; JAMA 2014;311:2414). Some centers prefer catheter-directed Rx (qv).
- **Moderate PE w/ large clot burden** (≥2 lobar arteries or main artery on CT or high prob VQ w/ ≥2 lobes w/ mismatch): low-dose lytic (50 mg if ≥50 kg or 0.5 mg/kg if <50 kg; for both 10 mg bolus → remainder over 2 h) ↓ pulm HTN w/ ≈ bleeding vs heparin alone; await further validation (Am J Cardiol 2013;111:273)
- **DVT:** consider if all are present (a) acute (<14 d) & extensive (eg, iliofemoral), (b) severe symptomatic swelling or ischemia (phlegmasia cerulea dolens), (c) catheter-directed Rx not available, and (d) low bleeding risk

Mechanical intervention
- **Catheter-directed therapy** (fibrinolytic & thrombus fragmentation/aspiration)
  Consider if extensive DVT (see above) and to ↓ post-thrombotic synd (Lancet 2012;379:31)
  Consider if PE w/ hemodyn. compromise or high risk & not candidate for systemic lysis or surgical thrombectomy (Circ 2011;124:2139). Preferred to systemic lytic by some centers.
  U/S-assisted → improves hemodynamics & RV fxn vs anticoag alone (EHJ 2015;36:597)
- **Thrombectomy:** if large, proximal PE + hemodynamic compromise + contra. to lysis; consider in experienced ctr if large prox. PE + RV dysfxn (J Thorac CV Surg 2005;129:1018)
- **IVC filter:** use instead of anticoagulation if latter contraindicated
  No benefit to adding to anticoag (including in submassive) (JAMA 2015;313:1627)
  Consider removable filter for temporary indications
  Complications: migration, acute DVT, ↑ risk of recurrent DVT & IVC obstruction (5–18%), which may lead to worsening LE sx (Archives 1992;152:1985)

Duration of full-intensity anticoagulation
- Superficial venous thrombosis: 4 wk
- 1st prox DVT or PE 2° reversible/time-limited risk factor or distal DVT: 3–6 mo
- 1st unprovoked prox DVT/ PE: ≥3 mo, then reassess; benefit to prolonged Rx (see below). Consider bleeding risk, Pt preference and intensity of extended Rx.
- 2nd VTE event or cancer: indefinite (or until cancer cured) (NEJM 1997;336:393 & 2003;348:1425)
- Does not appear that can rely on D-dimer testing to guide d/c (Annals 2015;162:27)

Extended antithrombotic strategies (JAMA 2015;314:72)
- After ≥6 mo of anticoag, following strategies have been compared w/ no extended Rx:
- Full-dose dabigatran, rivaroxaban, or apixaban: 80–90% ↓ recurrent VTE, 2–5× bleeding, but no signif excess in major bleeding (NEJM 2010;363:2499; 2013;368:699 & 709)
- Full-dose warfarin: 85% ↓ reduction in recurrent VTE (JAMA 2015;314:72)
- Low-intensity warfarin (INR 1.5–2.0): 64% ↓ reduction in recurrent VTE (NEJM 2003;348:1425)
- Low-intensity apixa (2.5 mg bid): 80% ↓ recur. VTE, w/o signif ↑ bleeding (NEJM 2013;368:699)
- Aspirin: 32% ↓ recurrent VTE (NEJM 2012;366:1959 & 367:1979)

Other therapeutic interventions
- Early ambulation
- For DVT: fitted graduated compression stockings (min 20–30 mmHg → 30–40 mmHg) for sx & to ↓ risk of postthrombotic synd (occurs in 23–60%; J Thromb Thrombolysis 2009;28:465)
- Leg elevation and exercise (use of calf muscle pump) also may be helpful
- Anticoag teaching: avoidance of high-risk activities, med alert bracelet, dietary instructions

Complications & prognosis
- Post-thrombotic syndrome (23–60%): thrombosis → injury to vein/valves → pain, edema, venous ulcers (J Thromb Thrombolysis 2009;28:465)
- Recurrent VTE: 1%/y (after 1st VTE) to 5%/y (after recurrent VTE)
  after only 6 mo of Rx: 5%/y & >10%/y, respectively
  predictors: abnl D-dimer 1 mo after d/c anticoag (NEJM 2006;355:1780); ⊕ U/S after 3 mo of anticoag (Annals 2002;137:955); thrombin generation >400 nM (JAMA 2006;296:397)
- Chronic thromboembolic PHT after acute PE ~3.8% (NEJM 2004;350:2257), consider thromboendarterectomy
- Mortality: ~10% for DVT and ~10–15% for PE at 3–6 mo (Circ 2008;117:1711)

PULMONARY HYPERTENSION (PHT)

PA mean pressure ≥25 mmHg at rest

Pathobiology (NEJM 2004;35:1655)

- Smooth muscle & endothelial cell proliferation; mutations in bone morphogenic protein receptor 2 (*BMPR2*) in ~50% familial & ~26% sporadic cases of IPAH (NEJM 2001;345:319)
- Imbalance between vasoconstrictors and vasodilators
   ↑ vasoconstrictors: thromboxane A_2 (TXA_2), serotonin (5-HT), endothelin-1 (ET-1)
   ↓ vasodilators: prostacyclin (PGI_2), nitric oxide (NO), vasoactive peptide (VIP)
- *In situ* thrombosis: ↑ TXA_2, 5-HT, PAI-1; ↓ PGI_2, NO, VIP, tissue plasminogen activator

Etiologies of Pulmonary Hypertension (Revised WHO Classification)	

Pulmonary arterial HTN (PAH) (group 1)	• Idiopathic (IPAH): mean age of onset 36 y (♂ older than ♀); ♀:♂ = ~2:1, usually mild ↑ in PAP
	• Familial (FPAH)
	• Associated conditions (APAH)
	  Connective tissue disorders: CREST, SLE, MCTD, RA, PM, Sjögren
	  Congenital: L→R shunts: ASD, VSD, PDA, 1° PHT of newborn
	  Portopulmonary HTN (? 2° vasoactive substances not filtered in ESLD; ≠ hepatopulmonary syndrome)
	  HIV; drugs & toxins: anorexic agents, rapeseed oil, L-tryptophan
	• Pulmonary veno-occlusive disease: ? 2° chemo, BMT; orthopnea, pl eff; nl PCWP; art vasodil. worsen pulm edema (AJRCCM 2000;162:1964)
	• Pulmonary capillary hemangiomatosis

Left heart disease (group 2)	• Left atrial or ventricular (diastolic or systolic) dysfunction • Left-sided valvular heart disease (eg, MS/MR > AS/AR) • Congenital: left-sided inflow/outflow obstruction, CMP
Lung diseases and/ or chronic hypoxemia (group 3)	• COPD • Alveolar hypoventilation (eg, NM disease) • ILD • Chronic hypoxemia (eg, high altitude) • Sleep apnea • Developmental abnormalities
Chronic thrombo-embolic dis (group 4)	• Prox or distal PEs; ~½ w/o clinical h/o PE (Circ 2014;130:508) • Nonthrombotic emboli (tumor, foreign body, parasites)
Miscellaneous (group 5)	• Sarcoidosis, histiocytosis X, LAM, schistosomiasis • Metab: thyroid, glycogen storage, Gaucher • Heme: chronic hemolytic anemia, myeloprolif d/o, splenectomy • Other: compression of pulm vessels (adenopathy, tumor, fibrosing mediastinitis, histoplasmosis, XRT); HHT (multifactorial)

(Circ 2013;62:25S)

Clinical manifestations

- Dyspnea, exertional syncope (hypoxia, ↓ CO), exertional chest pain (RV ischemia)
- Symptoms of R-sided CHF (eg, peripheral edema, RUQ fullness, abdominal distention)
- WHO class: I = asx w/ ordinary activity; II = sx w/ ord. activ; III = sx w/ min activ; IV = sx at rest

Physical exam

- PHT: prominent P_2, R-sided S_4, RV heave, PA tap & flow murmur, PR (Graham Steell), TR
- ± RV failure: ↑ JVP, hepatomegaly, peripheral edema

Diagnostic studies & workup (Circ 2014;130:1820)

- IPAH yearly incidence 1–2 per million, ∴ r/o 2° causes
- High-res chest CT: dil. & pruning of pulm arteries, ↑ RA and RV; r/o parenchymal lung dis.
- ECG: RAD, RBBB, RAE ("P pulmonale"), RVH (Se 55%, Sp 70%)
- PFTs: disproportionate ↓ D_{LCO}, mild restrictive pattern; r/o obstructive & restrict. lung dis.
- ABG & polysomnography: ↓ P_aO_2 and S_aO_2 (espec w/ exertion), ↓ P_aCO_2, ↑ A-a gradient; r/o hypoventilation and OSA
- TTE: ↑ RVSP (but estimate over/under by ≥10 mmHg in ½ of PHT Pts; Chest 2011;139:988)
   ↑ RA, RV (RV:LV area >1) and PA size; TR, PR
   ↑ RVSP → interventricular septum systolic flattening ("D" shape)
   ↑ RAP → interatrial septum bowing into LA
   ↓ RV systolic fxn: TAPSE (tricuspid annular plane systolic excursion) <1.6 cm; lateral-septal tissue-Doppler imaging disparity (reflecting relatively more systolic dysfxn of RV lateral wall vs septum, which is shared with LV)
   ↑ PA impedance → RVOT Doppler notching
   r/o LV dysfxn, MV or AoV disease, and congenital heart disease
- RHC: ↑ RA, RV, & PA pressures; ✓ L-sided pressures and for shunt
   if PAH: nl PCWP, ↑ transpulm gradient (mean PAP-PCWP >12–15), ↑ PVR, ± ↓ CO
   if 2° to L-heart disease: PCWP (or LVEDP) >15; if PVR nl → "passive PHT"; PVR >240 suggests mixed picture: if ↓ PCWP → ↓ PVR, then "reactive" PHT; if no Δ, then "fixed"

- CTA (large/med vessel), V/Q scan (small vessel to r/o CTEPH), ± pulmonary angiogram: r/o PE and chronic thromboembolic disease
- Vasculitis labs: ANA (~40% ⊕ in PAH), RF, anti-Scl-70, anticentromere, ESR
- LFTs & HIV: r/o portopulmonary and HIV-associated PAH
- 6-min walk test (6MWT) or cardiopulmonary exercise testing to establish fxnl capacity

Differentiating Left Heart Disease from Alternative PHT Etiologies		
Feature	Favors Left Heart Disease	Favors Alternative Etiology
History	Prior MI, CMP, AoV or MV disease, CV risk factors (HTN, diabetes), ↑ age	Family hx PHT, connective tissue disorder, pulm, liver or hematologic disease, HIV, h/o VTE
PEx	L-sided S3, S4 L-sided murmurs Displaced apical impulse Coarse rales	Cyanosis, clubbing Fine rales; signs of COPD Raynaud's, sclerodactyly, telangiectasia Splenomegaly, spider angiomata
ECG	Q waves, LVH, LBBB	Isolated RAE, RVH, $S_IQ_{III}T_{III}$ pattern
Echo	LV systolic or diastolic dysfxn LVH, ↑ LA size ≥Moderate MV or AoV disease	Isolated RV or RA enlargement Interventricular septum systolic flattening and/or interatrial septum bowing into LA ↓ RV systolic fxn
RHC	↑ L-sided filling pressures Abrupt ↑ PCWP (to >20–25) w/ exercise or volume loading	PCWP <15 mmHg Exercise PCWP <20–25 mmHg

Treatment (JACC 2013;62:25S & 2015;65:1976)

- Principles
  1) prevent and reverse vasoactive substance imbalance and vascular remodeling
  2) prevent RV failure: ↓ wall stress (↓ PVR, PAP, RV diam); ensure adeq. systemic DBP
- Supportive

  Oxygen: maintain S_aO_2 >90–92% (reduces vasoconstriction)

  Diuretics: ↓ RV wall stress and relieve RHF sx; gentle b/c RV is preload dependent

  Digoxin: control HR, ? counteract neg. inotropic effects CCB

  Dobutamine and inhaled NO or prostacyclin for decompensated PHT

  Anticoagulation: ↓ VTE risk of RHF; ? prevention of in situ microthrombi;

  ? mortality benefit even if in NSR, no RCTs (Circ 1984;70:580; Chest 2006;130:545)

  Supervised exercise training (Eur Respir J 2012;40:84)
- Vasodilators (right heart catheterization prior to initiation)

  acute vasoreactivity test: use inhaled NO, adenosine or prostacyclin to identify Pts likely to have a long-term response to oral CCB (⊕ vasoreactive response defined as ↓ PAP ≥10 mmHg to a level <40 mmHg with ↑ or stable CO); ~10% Pts are acute responders; no response → still candidates for other vasodilators (NEJM 2004;351:1425)

Vasoactive agents	Comments (data primarily in Group 1 PAH)
Oral CCB Nifedipine, diltiazem	If ⊕ acute vasoreactive test; <½ will be long-term responder (NYHA I/II & near-nl hemodynamics) & have ↓ mortality. Side effects: HoTN, lower limb edema (NEJM 1992;327:76; Circ 2005;111:3105).
IV Prostacyclin Epoprostenol (Flolan)	Vasodilation, ↓ plt agg, ↓ smooth muscle proliferation; benefits ↑ w/ time (? vascular remodeling). ↑ 6MWT, ↑ QoL, ↓ mortality. Side effects: HA, flushing, jaw/leg pain, abd cramps, nausea, diarrhea, catheter infxn (NEJM 1996;334:296 & 1998:338:273; Annals 2000;132:425).
Prostacyclin analogues Iloprost (inhaled) Treprostinil (IV, inh, SC) Beraprost (PO)	Same mechanism as prostacyclin IV, but easier to take, ↓ side effects, and w/o risk of catheter infxn, ↓ sx, ↑ 6MWT; trend to ↓ clinical events w/ iloprost but not treprostinil. Beraprost w/o sustained outcome improvement (n/a in U.S.) (NEJM 2002:347:322; AJRCCM 2002;165:800).
Endothelin receptor antagonists (ERAs) Bosentan, ambrisentan, macitentan	↓ Smooth muscle remodeling, vasodilation, ↓ fibrosis, ↓ sx, ↑ 6MWT, ↓ worsening PAH or need for prostanoids w/ trend for ↓ PAH mortality (w/ macitentan). Side effects: ↑ LFTs, headache, anemia, edema, teratogen (NEJM 2002:346:896; JACC 2005;46:529; Circ 2008;117:3010; NEJM 2013;369:809).
PDE-5 Inhibitor Sildenafil, tadalafil	↑ cGMP → vasodilation, ↓ smooth muscle proliferation, ↓ sx, ↑6MWT, no data on clinical outcomes. Low side-effect profile: HA, vision Δ's, sinus congestion (NEJM 2009;361:1864).
Soluble guanylate cyclase stimulator Riociguat	NO-independent ↑ cGMP → vasodilation, ↓ smooth muscle proliferation, ↓ sx, ↑ 6MWT in PAH; ↓ sx, ↓ PVR, ↑ 6MWT in CTEPH (NEJM 2013;369:319 & 330)

- Up front combination Rx (tadalafil + ambrisentan vs monotherapy): ↓ sx, ↓ NT-BNP, ↑ 6MWT, ↓ hospitalizations *(NEJM 2015;373:834)*
- Treat underlying causes of 2° PHT; can use vasodilators, although little evidence beyond riociguat use for CTEPH as described above
- Refractory PHT:
  balloon atrial septostomy: R→L shunt causes ↑ CO, ↓ S$_a$O$_2$, net ↑ tissue O$_2$ delivery
  lung transplant (single or bilateral); heart-lung needed if Eisenmenger physiology

Figure 1-7 Treatment of PAH (modified from *JACC* 2009;54:S78)

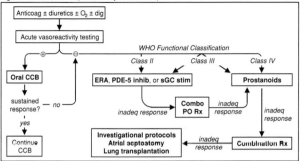

Management of ICU patient
- Avoid overly aggressive volume resuscitation
- Caution with vasodilators if any L-sided dysfunction
- May benefit from inotropes/chronotropes
- Mechanical RV support (RVAD, ECMO) *(Circ 2015;132:526)*
- Consider fibrinolysis if acute, refractory decompensation (eg, TPA 100 mg over 2 h)

Prognosis
- Median survival after dx ~2.8 y; PAH (all etiologies): 2-y 66%, 5-y 48% *(Chest 2004;126:78-S)*
- Poor prognostic factors: clinical evidence of RV failure, rapidly progressive sx, WHO (modified NYHA) class IV, 6MWT <300 m, peak VO$_2$ <10.4 mL/kg/min, ↑ RA or RV or RV dysfxn, RA >20 or CI <2.0, ↑ BNP *(Chest 2006;129:1313)*
- Lung transplant: 1-y survival 66–75%; 5-y survival 45–55% *(Chest 2004;126:63-S)*

BRADYCARDIA AND AV BLOCK

BRADYCARDIAS

Sinus bradycardia (SB) (*NEJM* 2000;342:703)
- Etiologies: **meds** (incl βB, CCB, amio, Li, dig), ↑ **vagal tone** (incl. in athletes, sleep, IMI), **metabolic** (hypoxia, sepsis, myxedema, hypothermia, ↓ glc), OSA, ↑ ICP
- Treatment: if no sx, none; atropine, β₁ agonists or long-term permanent pacing if sx
- Most common cause of sinus pause is *blocked premature atrial beat*

Sick sinus syndrome (SSS)
- Features may include: periods of unprovoked SB, SA arrest, paroxysms of SB and atrial tachyarrhythmias ("tachy-brady" syndrome), chronotropic incompetence w/ ETT
- Treatment: meds alone usually fail (adeq. control of tachy → unacceptable brady); usually need **combination of meds** (βB, CCB, dig) for tachy & **PPM** for brady

Pseudobradycardia
- Intermittent PVCs (with low stroke volume and hence low pulse wave) followed by compensatory pause can cause ascertainment of HR by palpation of radial pulse to be artifactually low

---

AV BLOCK AND AV DISSOCIATION

AV Block	
Type	**Features**
1°	Prolonged PR (>200 ms), all atrial impulses conducted (1:1)
2° Mobitz I (Wenckebach)	Progressive ↑ PR until impulse not conducted (→ "grouped beating") Due to **AV node** conduction delay: ischemia (IMI), inflammation (myocarditis, MV surgery), high vagal tone (athletes), drug-induced QRS duration most often normal AVB usually worsens w/ carotid sinus massage, improves w/ atropine & exercise Often paroxysmal/nocturnal/asymptomatic; no Rx required
2° Mobitz II	Occasional or repetitive blocked impulses w/ consistent PR interval. Nb, do not confuse with APBs in bigeminal pattern; to dx AVB, atrial rate should be *regular* and P waves should be the *same*. Due to **His-Purkinje** conduction delay: ischemia (AMI), degeneration of conduction system, infiltrative disease, inflammation/valve surgery QRS duration often prolonged AVB usually improves w/ carotid sinus massage, worsens w/ atropine & exercise (both of which should be *avoided* if dx suspected) Risk of progression to 3° AVB. Zoll at bedside when recognized; temp pacing wire or PPM often required.
3° (complete)	No AV conduction, with ventricular rhythm slower than atrial rhythm Escape, if present is regular and can be narrow (jxnal) or wide (vent.) Urgent temporary pacing as bridge to permanent pacing is appropriate in most scenarios, especially when syncope present

Nb, if 2:1 block, cannot distinguish type I vs II 2° AVB (no chance to observe PR prolongation); usually categorize based on other ECG & clinical data. High-grade AVB usually refers to block of ≥2 successive impulses. All categories above assume SR in atrium, criteria do not apply during rapid atrial rates, such as in atrial flutter or tachycardia.

AV dissociation
- *Default:* slowing of SA node allows subsidiary pacemaker (eg, AV junction) to take over
- *Usurpation:* acceleration of subsidiary pacemaker (eg, AV junctional tach, VT)
- *3° AV block:* atrial pacemaker unable to capture ventricles, subsidiary pacemaker emerges; distinguish from *isorhythmic dissociation* (A ≈ V rate, some P waves nonconducting)

Temporary pacing wires
- Consider w/ bradycardia with hemodyn instability or unstable escape rhythm when perm pacer not readily available. Risks: RV perf, VT, PTX, CHB if existing LBBB, etc.
- Consider instead of PPM for sx bradycardia due to reversible cause (βB/CCB O/D, Lyme, myocarditis, SBE, s/p cardiac surgery/trauma), TdP, acute MI (sx brady, high-grade AVB)

PALPITATIONS

Etiologies
- PACs; PVCs; SVT, AF, VT, respiratory sinus arrhythmia; pauses; noncardiac

Workup
- History: duration & frequency; initiating & aggravating factors: exercise, alcohol, stimulants (caffeine, pseudoephedrine, other prescription & recreational drugs); h/o presyncope or syncope; FHx of arrhythmia, CMP, SCD
- Structural evaluation w/ echo; consider ETT if exercise-induced or other RF; TFTs
- Ambulatory cardiac monitoring: *must monitor during symptoms to diagnose!*
  Holter (worn continuously): if sx typically occur within a 24–48-hr period
  Looping event monitor (worn continuously): if sx fleeting
  Nonlooping event monitor (put on during sx): if rarer episodes lasting minutes

Treatment (for SVT and VT, see respective sections)
- Simple ectopy in structurally normal heart: reassurance, βB, CCB. If refractory, frequent sx with poor QoL, antiarrhythmic drug, such as flecainide, can be tried in consultation w/ electrophysiologist. Rarely catheter ablation for frequent PVCs.
- If NICM and >13% PVCs, elim of ectopy w/ catheter ablation can significantly ↑ EF (*JACC* 2013;62:1195). However, risk of *developing* CMP due to frequent PVCs not established.

SUPRAVENTRICULAR TACHYCARDIAS (SVTs)

*Arise above the ventricles, ∴ **narrow QRS** unless aberrant conduction or pre-excitation*

Common Etiologies of SVT (NEJM 2006;354:1039 & 2012;367:1438)		
	Type	**Features**
Atrial	Sinus tachycardia (ST)	Caused by pain, fever, hypovolemia, hypoxia, anemia, anxiety, β-agonists, etc.
	Atrial tachycardia (AT)	Originate at site in atria other than SA node. Seen w/ CAD, COPD, ↑ catechols, EtOH, dig.
	Multifocal atrial tachycardia (MAT)	↑ automaticity at multiple sites in the atria. Seen with underlying pulmonary disease.
	Atrial flutter (AFL)	Macroreentry, usually w/in right atrium
	Atrial fibrillation (AF)	Chaotic atrial activation and rapid, irregular bombardment of AVN
AV Jxn	AV nodal reentrant tach (AVNRT)	Reentrant circuit using dual pathways w/in AVN
	AV reciprocating tachycardia (AVRT)	Reentrant circuit using AVN antegrade and accessory pathway retrograde. When in sinus rhythm may show pre-excitation (WPW) or not (concealed accessory pathway)
	Paroxysmal junctional reciprocating tachycardia (PJRT)	Reentry using AVN & slowly conducting concealed posterosept acc path. More common in peds, at times w/ tachy-induced CMP.
	Nonparoxysmal junctional tachycardia (NPJT)	↑ jxnal automaticity. May see retrograde P's & AV dissoc. A/w myo/endocarditis, cardiac surg, IMI, dig.

Diagnosis of SVT Type (NEJM 2006;354:1039 & 2012;367:1438)	
Onset	Abrupt on/off argues against sinus tachycardia
Rate	Not dx as most can range from 140–250 bpm, *but:* ST usually <150; AFL often conducts 2:1 → vent. rate 150; AVNRT & AVRT usually >150
Rhythm	Irregular → AF, AFL w/ variable block, or MAT

P wave	Long RP: ST (P same as sinus), AT, MAT (≥3 morphologies), PJRT
	Short RP, P inverted in inf. leads → *retrograde* atrial activation via AVN
	  AVNRT: buried in or distort terminal portion of QRS (pseudo-RSR′ in V₁)
	  AVRT: slightly after QRS (RP interval >100 ms favors AVRT vs AVNRT)
	  NPJT: either no P wave or retrograde P similar to AVNRT
	Fibrillation or no P waves → AF
	Saw-toothed "F" waves (best seen in inferior leads & V₁) → AFL

Response to vagal stim. or adenosine	Slowing of HR often seen with ST, AF, AFL, AT, whereas reentrant rhythms (AVNRT, AVRT) may abruptly terminate (classically w/ P wave after last QRS) or no response. Occ AT may terminate. AFL & AF → ↑ AV block → unmasking of "F" waves or fibrillation

Short RP: P wave closer to preceding than following QRS (ie, RP < PR). Long RP: P wave closer to following than preceding QRS (ie, PR < RP).

Figure 1-8 Approach to SVT

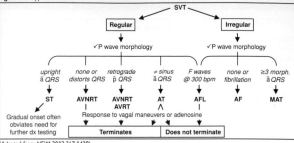

(Adapted from *NEJM* 2012;367:1438)

Treatment of SVT		
Rhythm	**Acute treatment**	**Long-term treatment**
Unstable	**Cardioversion** per ACLS	n/a
ST	Treat underlying stressor(s)	n/a
AT	βB, CCB or amiodarone; ? vagal maneuvers or adenosine	βB or CCB, ± antiarrhythmics, possibly radiofrequency ablation (RFA)
AVNRT or AVRT	**Vagal maneuvers** **Adenosine** (caution in AVRT*) **CCB** or βB	*For AVNRT (see next section for AVRT):* **RFA.** CCB or βB (chronic or prn) ± Class IC antiarrhythmics (if nl heart)
NPJT	**CCB, βB,** amiodarone	Rx underlying dis. (eg, dig tox, ischemia)
AF	**βB, CCB, digoxin, AAD**	See "Atrial Fibrillation"
AFL	**βB, CCB, digoxin, AAD**	RFA; βB or CCB ± antiarrhythmics
MAT	CCB or βB if tolerated	Treat underlying disease process AVN ablation + PPM if refractory to meds

*Avoid adenosine & nodal agents if accessory pathway + preexcited tachycardia, see below (*JACC* 2003;42:1493)

- *Catheter ablation:* high overall success rate (AFL/AVNRT ~95%, AVRT ~90%, AF ~80%) Complications: stroke, MI, bleeding, perforation, conduction block (*JAMA* 2007;290:2768)

ACCESSORY PATHWAYS (WOLFF-PARKINSON-WHITE)

Definitions
- **Accessory pathway** (bypass tract) of conducting myocardium connecting atria & ventricles, allowing impulses to bypass normal AVN delay
- **Preexcitation (WPW) pattern:** ↓ PR interval, ↑ QRS width w/ δ wave (slurred onset, *can be subtle*), ST & Tw abnl (can mimic old IMI); *only seen w/ pathways that conduct antegrade* (if pathway only conducts retrograde then ECG will be normal during SR; "concealed" bypass tract) PAC can exaggerate preexcitation if AV node conduction slowed
- **WPW syndrome:** accessory pathway + paroxysmal tachycardia

Classic tachycardias of WPW
- **Orthodromic AVRT:** *narrow-complex* SVT (typically), conducting ↓ AVN & ↑ accessory pathway; requires retrograde conduction & ∴ can occur w/ concealed bypass tracts
- **Antidromic AVRT** (less common): *wide-complex* regular tachycardia, conducting ↓ accessory pathway & ↑ AVN. Can meet many ECG morphology criteria for VT. Requires antegrade conduction and ∴ should see WPW pattern during SR.
- **AF** w/ rapid conduction down accessory pathway; ∴ wide-complex irregular SVT; requires antegrade conduction; ∴ should see WPW pattern in SR. Rarely can degenerate into VF.

Treatment
- **AVRT:** vagal, βB; caution w/ adenosine (can precip. AF); have defibrillator ready
- **AF/AFL** w/ conduction down accessory pathway: need to Rx arrhythmia *and* ↑ pathway refractoriness; use **procainamide, ibutilide,** or DCCV; avoid CCB & βB, dig/adenosine (can ↓ refractoriness of pathway → ↑ vent. rate → VF)
- **Long term:** Rx sx tachycardias w/ RFA, antiarrhythmics (IA, IC) if not candidate for RFA. Consider RFA if asx but AVRT or AF inducible on EPS (*NEJM* 2003;349:1803) or if rapid conduction possible (✓ w/ EPS if preexcitation persists despite exercise testing). Risk of SCD related to how short RR interval is in AF and # of accessory pathways present. Exercise testing to look for loss of pre-excitation can be used as a proxy for short RR interval in AF: if pathway still present at peak exercise, more concerning.

ATRIAL FIBRILLATION

Classification (*Circ 2014;130:2071*)
- **Paroxysmal** (terminates spontaneously or w/ Rx w/in 7 d) vs **persistent** (sustained >7 d) vs **long-standing persistent** (>1 y) vs **permanent** (no plan to restore or maintain SR)
- **Nonvalvular** (AF absent rheumatic MS, prosthetic valve or mitral valve repair) vs **valvular**
- **Lone AF** = age <60 y and w/o clinical or echo evidence of cardiac disease (including HTN)

Pathophysiology
- Disorganized atrial electrical activity → ineffective atrial mechanical contraction
- For paroxysmal AF, >90% triggered by rapid firing in pulmonary veins (*NEJM 1998;339:659*)

Epidemiology and etiologies (*Annals 2008;149:ITC5-2*)
- 1–2% of pop. has AF (8% of elderly); lifetime risk 25%; mean age at presentation ~75 y
- Acute (up to 50% w/o identifiable cause)
    Cardiac: HF, myo/pericarditis, ischemia/MI, hypertensive crisis, cardiac surgery
    Pulmonary: acute pulmonary disease or hypoxia (eg, COPD flare, PNA), PE, OSA
    Metabolic: high catecholamine states (stress, infection, postop, pheo), thyrotoxicosis
    Drugs: alcohol ("holiday heart"), cocaine, amphetamines, theophylline, caffeine
    Neurogenic: subarachnoid hemorrhage, ischemic stroke
- Chronic: ↑ age, HTN, ischemia, valve dis. (MV, TV, AoV), CMP, hyperthyroidism, obesity

Evaluation
- H&P, ECG, CXR, TTE (LA size, thrombus, valves, LV fxn, pericardium), K, Mg, FOBT before anticoag, TFTs; r/o MI not necessary unless other ischemic sx

Figure 1-9 Approach to acute AF

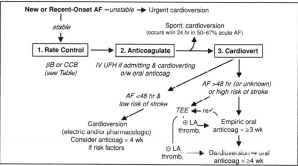

(Adapted from *NEJM 2004;351:2408; JACC 2006;48:e149*)

Rate control
- If sx, goal HR <80; if asx & EF >40%, goal HR <110 at rest (*NEJM 2010;362:1363*)
- AV node ablation + PPM if pharmacologic Rx inadequate (*NEJM 2001;344:1043; 2002;346:2062*)

Rate Control for AF				
Agent		**Acute (IV)**	**Maint. (PO)**	**Comments**
CCB	Verapamil	5–10 mg over 2′ may repeat in 30′	120–360 mg/d in divided doses	↓ BP (Rx w/ Ca gluc) Can worsen HF
	Diltiazem	0.25 mg/kg over 2′ may repeat after 15′ 5–15 mg/h infusion	120–360 mg/d in divided doses	Preferred if severe COPD Can ↑ dig levels
βB	Metoprolol	2.5–5 mg over 2′ may repeat q5′ × 3	25–100 mg bid or tid	↓ BP (Rx w/ glucagon) Preferred if CAD Risks: HF & bronchospas.
Digoxin* (onset >30 min)		0.25 mg q2h up to 1.5 mg	0.125–0.375 mg qd (adj for CrCl)	Consider in HF or low BP Poor exertional HR ctrl
Amiodarone		300 mg over 1 h → 0.5–1 mg/min × 24 h	100–200 mg QD	Consider in HF or low BP Long-term potential tox

IV βB, CCB and digoxin ***contraindicated*** if evidence of WPW (ie, pre-excitation or WCT) since may facilitate conduction down accessory pathway leading to VF; ∴ use procainamide, ibutilide or amiodarone
*Many meds incl. amio, verapamil, quinidine, propafenone, macrolides & azole antifungals ↑ digoxin levels.

Cardioversion

- Consider pharm or electrical cardioversion w/ 1st AF episode or if sx;
  if AF >48 h, 2–5% risk stroke w/ cardioversion (*pharmacologic or electric*)
  ∴ either TEE to r/o thrombus or ensure therapeutic anticoagulation for ≥3 wk prior
  if need to cardiovert urgently, anticoagulate acutely (eg, IV UFH)
- Likelihood of success ∝ AF duration & atrial size; correct precip. (eg, vol status, thyroid)
- Consider pre-Rx w/ antiarrhythmic drugs (eg, ibutilide), espec if 1st cardioversion fails
- For pharmacologic cardioversion, class III and IC drugs have best proven efficacy
- If SR returns (spont. or w/ Rx), atria may be *mech. stunned;* also, high risk of recurrent AF
  over next 3 mo. ∴ **Anticoag postcardioversion ≥4 wk** (? unless <48 h and low risk).

Rhythm control (Lancet 2012;379:648; Circ 2014;130:2071)

- No clear survival benefit or ↓ stroke risk vs rate control (NEJM 2002;347:1825 & 2008;358:2667)
- Consider if *symptomatic* w/ rate control (eg, heart failure), difficult to control rate, or
  tachycardia-mediated cardiomyopathy

Antiarrhythmic Drugs (AAD) for AF (Circ 2011;123:104 & 2012;125:381; EHJ 2012;33:2719)			
Agent	Conversion	Maintenance	Comments
III Amiodarone	5–7 mg/kg IV over 30–60′ → 1 mg/min, 10 g load	200–400 mg qd (most effective AAD for SR)	↑ QT, but TdP rare. Low rate of acute conversion. May convert wks after load, ∴ attention to anticoag. Pulm, liver, thyroid toxicity ✓ PFTs, LFTs, TFTs. Potentiates warfarin, ∴ ↓ warfarin by ~50%
Dronedarone	n/a	400 mg bid	↓ side effects but also ↓ effic. c/w amio; contraindic. in perm AF or sx HF / ↓ EF; risk of liver toxicity
Ibutilide	1 mg IV over 10′ may repeat × 1	n/a	Contraindic. if ↓ K or ↑ QT ↑ QT, 3–8% risk of TdP Mg 1–2 g IV to ↓ risk TdP Lasts 4–6 h
Dofetilide	500 mcg PO bid	500 mcg mg bid	↑ QT, ↑ risk of TdP; renal adj
Sotalol	n/a	80–160 mg bid	✓ for ↓ HR, ↑ QT; renal adj
IC Flecainide	300 mg PO × 1	100–150 mg bid	PreRx w/ AVN blocker *Contraindic. if structural or ischemic heart disease*
Propafenone	600 mg PO × 1	150–300 mg tid	
IA Procainamide	10–15 mg/kg IV over 1 h	n/a	↓ BP; ↑ QT ± PreRx w/ AVN blocker
Underlying disease		**Maintenance AAD of choice**	
None or minimal (incl HTN w/o LVH)		class IC ("pill in pocket"), sotalol, dronedarone	
HTN w/ LVH		amiodarone	
CAD		sotalol, dofetilide, amiodarone, dronedarone	
HF		amiodarone, dofetilide	

Radiofrequency ablation (JAMA 2015;314:278)

- **Rationale:** Controlling triggers in pulmonary veins can control AF when little atrial scar present. As progress to persistent and permanent, LA substrate more complex due to scarring and is likely harder to ablate with pulmonary vein isolation alone.
- **Indication:** reasonable alternative to AAD in structurally normal heart
- **Approach:** for paroxysmal AF, circumferential pulm. vein isolation done via ablation in LA myocardium (ablation in PVs causes stenosis) w/ ~80% success (Lancet 2012;380:1509).
  In AF w/o ↑↑ LA or ↓ EF, RFA still superior to AAD, but lower success rate w/ AF recurring in ~1/2 over 2 y and 2nd RFA often required to prevent LA flutter (NEJM 2012;367:1587; JAMA 2014;311:692). Utility of upfront additional lines of block unclear (NEJM 2015;372:1812).
- Often performed on uninterrupted/minimally interrupt warfarin or Xa inhib (Circ 2014;129:1688)
- **Risks and complications**
  ↑ arrhythmia & pericarditis during healing post ablation
  left atrial flutters may persist and need additional "touch up" ablation
  rarer complications (1–2%): stroke, tamponade, phrenic nerve injury, PV stenosis,
  LA-esophageal/mediastinal communication (~3 wk after procedure, severe dysphagia,
  fever, CNS signs of thromboembolism; dx w/ CT scan or barium study, *no TEE*;
  emergent thoracic surgery)
- Surgical "maze" procedure (70–95% success rate) option if undergoing cardiac surgery

Oral anticoagulation *(Circ 2014;130:2071; JAMA 2015;313:1950)*

- *All valvular AF* (ie, rheum MS, valve prosthesis or repair), as stroke risk very high
- Nonvalvular AF (NVAF): stroke risk ~4.5%/y, but varies depending on patient; anticoagulation → 68% ↓ stroke but carries risk of bleeding; ∴ use a risk score to guide Rx
- **CHA₂DS₂-VASc:** CHF (1 point), **H**TN (1), **A**ge ≥75 y (2), DM (1), **S**troke/TIA (2), **V**ascular disease (MI, PAD, or aortic plaque) (1), **A**ge 65–74 y (1), ♀ **S**ex category (1) annual risk of stroke *(Lancet 2012;379:648)*: at low level, ~1% per point: 0 → ~0%, 1 → 1.3%, 2 → 2.2%, 3 → 3.2%, 4 → 4.0%; at higher scores, risk ↑↑ (5 → 6.7%, ≥6 → ≥10%)
- Anticoagulation recommendations: **score ≥2 → anticoagulate**
  score 1 → consider anticoagulation or antiplatelet Rx (? latter reasonable if risk factor 65–74 y, vasc disease or ♀) or no Rx
  score 0 → reasonable to not anticoagulate
- **HAS-BLED** *(Chest 2010;138:1093)*
  HTN (1 point if >160 mmHg), **A**bnl renal/liver fxn (1 for each), **S**troke (1), **B**leeding hx or predisposition (eg, anemia), **L**abile INR (time in therapeutic range <60%), **E**lderly (eg, age >65, frailty), **D**rugs/alcohol concom (1 point for antiplt or NSAID; 1 for alcohol)
  ≥3 → ↑ risk for bleeding, ∴ consider closer monitoring or different drug/dose selection
- Special situations in Pts w/ indication for anticoagulation:
  plan for rhythm control: continue anticoagulation
  Pt refuses anticoag: ASA + clopi or, even less effective, ASA alone *(NEJM 2009;360:2066)*
  underwent PCI: ? Rx w/ anticoagulant & clopidogrel, omit ASA *(Lancet 2013;381:1107)*
- **Anticoagulant options:** factor Xa or direct thrombin inhib (NVAF only) or **warfarin** (INR 2–3; w/ UFH bridge if high risk of stroke)
- Periop rate of arterial embolization in AF (w/o mech valve) <0.5%; ∅ benefit to bridging anticoag w/ LMWH & ↑ bleeding c/w stopping warf 5 d before *(NEJM 2015;373:823)*

Novel Oral Anticoagulants for Nonvalvular AF		
Anticoag	**Dosing**	**Efficacy & safety vs warfarin**
Dabigatran (Direct thromb inhib)	150 mg bid (110 not avail in U.S.) (75 mg bid if CrCl 15–30)	150 mg: ↓ ischemic stroke & ICH 110 mg: ≈ ischemic stroke & ↓ major bleed/ICH Risks: GI side effects, ↑ MI c/w warfarin
Rivaroxaban (FXa inhib)	20 mg qd (15 mg qd if CrCl 15–50) w/ pm meal	≈ ischemic stroke & ↓ major bleed incl ICH
Apixaban (FXa inhib)	5 mg bid (2.5 mg bid if ≥2 risks: ≥80 y, <60 kg, Cr ≥1.5 mg/dL)	≈ ischemic stroke & ↓ major bleed incl ICH, 11% ↓ death In Pts felt not cand for warfarin, apixa 55% ↓ stroke w/o ↑ bleed vs ASA alone.
Edoxaban (Fxa inhib)	60 mg qd if CrCl 51–95 (30 mg if CrCl 15–50) (30/15 mg regimen not available in U.S.)	60/30 mg: ≈ ischemic stroke & ↓ major bleed incl ICH, 14% ↓ CV death 30/15 mg: ↑ ischemic stroke & ↓↓ major bleed incl ICH, 15% ↓ CV death

- Rapid onset (w/in several hrs) and offset. Consequently do not need to bridge when starting. However, missing 1 dose could lead to inadequate protection.
- No monitoring required
- Require dose adjustment based on renal fxn, which should be monitored while on drug
- Difficult to reverse if bleeding. Prothrombin complex concentrate or recombinant FVIIa needed. Dabi can be reversed w/ idarucizumab (Ab frag; *NEJM 2015;373:511*).

(NEJM 2009;361:1139; 2011;364:806; 365:883 & 981; 2013;369:2063; Lancet 2014;383:955)

Nonpharmacologic stroke prevent *(ACC/HRS/SCAI 2015 Overview, JACC 2015)*
- Percutaneous occlusion of left atrial appendage (LAA) w/ watchman device (nitinol cage w/ polyethylene membrane). Postprocedure: warfarin × ~45 d followed by clopi × ~4.5 mo and ASA lifelong. In NVAF w/ CHADS₂ ≥1-2, c/w warfarin, ≈ stroke (↓ hemorrhagic, ↑ ischemic), ↓ bleeding (↑ procedural, ↓ non-proc), ↓ CV death *(JACC 2015;65:2614)*. Does not address issue of high-risk anticoag Pt w/ *existing* LAA thrombus.
- Epicardial snare to ligate LAA (lariat device). High rate of initial technical success *(JACC 2013;62:108)*, but long-term clinical outcomes & safety to be defined.
- Surgical LAA resection reasonable if another indication for cardiac surgery. Resection superior to ligation, which can recanalize.

Atrial flutter
- Macroreentrant atrial loop typically involving cavotricuspid isthmus (usually counter-clockwise w/ flutter waves ⊖ in inf leads & ⊕ in V₁, but can be clockwise).
- Risk of stroke similar to that of AF; ∴ same mandate for stroke prevention.
- Ablation of cavotricuspid isthmus has 95% success rate w/ only 0.5% complication rate. Pts remain at risk for atrial fibrillation.

Etiologies (Lancet 2012;380:1520)
- **Ventricular tachycardia (VT):** accounts for 80% of WCT in unselected population
- **SVT conducted with aberrancy:** either fixed BBB, rate-dependent BBB (usually RBBB), conduction via an accessory pathway or atrially triggered ventricular pacing

Monomorphic ventricular tachycardia (MMVT)
- All beats look similar; predominantly upward in V_1 = RBBB-type vs downward = LBBB-type
- Most commonly in obviously *structurally abnormal heart*: prior MI (scar); **CMP**
  mechanism is most commonly re-entry around areas of electrically silent scar tissue with slow myocardial conduction through adjacent areas of surviving myocytes
  focal arrhythmias also occur (RVOT, Ao root, fascicles, papillary muscles)
  re-entry utilizing the Purkinje system is also seen (Bundle Branch Reentry); "typical" form occurs in Pts w/ LBBB in sinus and VT w/ very similar morphology to sinus
- May occur in *apparently nl heart that is actually diseased:*
  Arrhythmogenic (RV) CMP (ACM, qv): incomplete RBBB, ε wave (terminal notch in QRS) & TWI in V_1–V_3 on resting ECG, LBBB-type VT; dx w/ MRI (Lancet 2009;373:1289)

  V_2 Epsilon

  subtle HCMP; sarcoid; myocarditis (incl giant cell); anom coronary
- In structurally *normal heart* w/ nl resting ECG (prog generally good):
  RVOT VT: LBBB-type VT w/ inferior axis; often seen immediately after exercise; can suppress with CCB or βB or ablate
  idiopathic LV VT: RBBB-type VT w/ superior axis; responds to verapamil or can ablate

Polymorphic ventricular tachycardia (PMVT)
- QRS morphology and/or axis changes from beat to beat
- Etiologies: **ischemia; CMP**
  torsades de pointes (TdP = "twisting of the points," PMVT + ↑ QT): ↑ QT *acquired* (meds, lytes, stroke; see "ECG") w/ risk ↑ w/ ↓ HR, freq PVCs (pause dependent) or *congenital* (K/Na channelopathies) w/ resting Tw abnl & TdP triggered by sympathetic stimulation (eg, exercise, emotion, sudden loud noises) (Lancet 2008;372:750)
  Brugada syndrome (Na channelopathy): ♂ > ♀; pseudo-RBBB w/ STE in V_1–V_3 (provoked w/ class IA or IC) on resting ECG

  catecholaminergic (CPVT): familial; mutations in ryanodine receptor or calsequestrin 2; presents during emotional or physical stress

Diagnostic clues that favor VT (assume until proven otherwise)
- **Prior MI, CHF** or **LV dysfxn** best predictors (90%) that WCT is VT (Am J Med 1998;84:53)
- Hemodynamics and rate do *not* reliably distinguish VT from SVT
- MMVT is regular, but may have initial "warmup period" and may be slightly irregular (as compared w/ SVT, which is extremely regular);
  grossly irregularly irregular rhythm suggests PMVT or AF w/ aberrancy
- More the QRS morphology is like QRS morphology in SR, more likely SVT
- ECG features that favor VT (Circ 1991;83:1649; EHJ 2007;28:589)
  AV dissociation (independent P waves, capture or fusion beats) proves VT;
  physical exam correlates: variable S_1 and cannon a waves on JVP
  very wide QRS (>140 ms in RBBB-type or >160 in LBBB-type)
  extreme axis deviation; RBBB-type w/ LAD; LBBB-type w/ RAD; shift in axis >40°; initial R wave in aVR
  QRS morphology atypical for BBB
  RBBB-type: absence of tall R' (or presence of monophasic R) in V_1, r/S ratio <1 in V_6
  LBBB-type: onset to nadir >60–100 ms in V_1, q wave in V_6
  longest RS interval in any precordial lead >100 ms and R wider than S
  ratio of voltage Δ in initial 40 msec to Δ in terminal 40 ms ≤1
  concordance (QRS in all precordial leads w/ same pattern/direction)

Acute management
- If stable: conscious sedation & sync cardioversion; if unstable (↓ BP, angina, ΔMS, HF): emergent cardioversion; if pulseless → ACLS w/ CPR & cardioversion
- Refractory: consider amiodarone, procainamide, and lidocaine (if suspect ischemia)
- If suspect PPM-mediated tachycardia → place magnet (switches device to VOO or DOO)
- If ICD: should deliver Rx, but do not rely on for VT resolution. If stable, can interrogate ICD. If repeated, appropriate & successful shocks → antiarrhythmics to suppress arrhythmia. If repeated shocks (approp or inapprop) w/o arrhythmia term → disable device (magnet).

Long-term management (JACC 2006;48:1064)
- Workup: **echo** to √ LV fxn, **cath** or **stress test** to r/o ischemia, ? MRI and/or RV bx to look for infiltrative CMP or ARVC, ? **EP study** to assess inducibility

- **ICD:** 2° prevention after documented VT/VF arrest (unless due to reversible cause)
  1° prev. if high risk, eg, EF <30–35%, ACM, Brugada, certain LQTS, severe HCM. See "Cardiac Rhythm Management Devices." ? Wearable vest if reversible etiology while waiting for ICD (*Circ* 2013;127:854).
  Antitachycardia pacing (ATP = burst pacing faster than VT) can terminate VT w/o shock
- **Meds:** βB, antiarrhythmics (eg, amio, mexiletine) to suppress VT, which could trigger shock
- If med a/w TdP → QT >500 ±VPBs: d/c med, replete K, give Mg, ± pacing (*JACC* 2010;55:934)
- **Radiofrequency ablation** if isolated VT focus or if recurrent VT triggering ICD firing; ablation before ICD implantation ↓ discharge rate by 40% (*Lancet* 2010;375:31)

SUDDEN CARDIAC DEATH (SCD)

Definition
- Sudden cessation of cardiac activity with hemodynamic collapse
- Technically sudden cardiac arrest (SCA) or "aborted SCD" if resuscitated
- Frequently due to sustained VT/VF

Etiologies
- **Coronary artery disease** (~60–70%)
  acute ischemia: ACS; spasm; congenital coronary artery anomaly
  scar from prior MI
- **Structurally abnormal heart or vasculature** (~10–15%)
  cardiomyopathy: DCM, HCM, ACM; myocarditis
  valvular heart disease
  myocardial rupture, tamponade, Ao dissection
  PE
- **Apparently structurally normal heart** (~10–15%)
  LQTS (acquired or congenital); Brugada syndrome; catecholaminergic polymorphic VT
  ACM or infiltrative cardiomyopathy
  Wolff-Parkinson-White (typically w/ antegrade conduction of AF → VF)
  complete heart block
  commotio cordis (*NEJM* 1995;333:337)

Precipitants
- Ischemia
- Drugs: antiarrhythmics, QT-prolonging, diuretics
- Electrolytes (usually not sufficient to cause SCD; always search for underlying cause)

Workup (*JACC* 2006;48:1064)
- Hx (usually very limited): may have had prodrome c/w ACS or HF; PMH; meds; FHx
- Exam: signs of cardiovascular disease
- ECG: ischemia, infarction, conduction block, QT, pre-excitation, abnormal V_1–V_3 (eg, pseudo-RBBB + STE, ε wave + TWI), LVH
- Echocardiogram; MRI if echo unrevealing and no other obvious cause
- Coronary angiography (? or CT angio)
  if STE or ? chest pain prodrome, urgent angio (unless poor neurologic prognosis)
  even w/o STE, 33–40% will have evidence of acute occlusion (*NEJM* 1997;336:1629 & *JACC Intv* 2015;8:1031)
- EP study (qv) if above workup unrevealing, programmed stimulation to look for accessory pathway, drug infusions to provoke arrhythmia from CPVT, LQTS, Brugada
- Exercise testing to provoke CPVT or assess resolution of pre-excitation to risk stratify WPW
- If genetic or unexplained SCD, evaluation of family members

SYNCOPE

Definition
- Sudden transient loss of consciousness due to global cerebral hypoperfusion
- If CPR or cardioversion required, then SCD (qv) and not syncope (different prognosis)
- Presyncope = prodrome of light-headedness without LOC

Epidemiology
- Incidence ↑ w/ age, particularly above 70 y; similar in men & women
- Lifetime incidence ~1 in 3

Etiologies (NEJM 2002;347:878; JACC 2006;47:473; EHJ 2009;30:2631)
- **Neurocardiogenic** (a.k.a. vasovagal, ~25%; NEJM 2005;352:1004)
  ↑ sympathetic tone → vigorous contraction of LV → mechanoreceptors in LV trigger ↑ vagal tone (hyperactive Bezold-Jarisch reflex) → ↓ HR (cardioinhibitory) and/or ↓ BP (vasodepressor)
  cough, deglutition, defecation, & micturition → ↑ vagal tone and thus can be precipitants
  carotid sinus hypersensitivity is a related disorder w/ an exaggerated vagal resp to carotid massage
- **Cardiovascular** (~20%, more likely in men than women)
  Arrhythmia (15%): challenging to dx as often transient
    Bradyarrhythmias: SSS, high-grade AV block (Stokes-Adams attack), ⊖ chronotropes, PPM malfunction
    Tachyarrhythmias: VT, SVT (syncope rare unless structural heart disease or WPW)
  Mechanical (5%)
    Endocardial/Valvular: AS, MS, PS, prosthetic valve thrombosis, atrial myxoma
    Myocardial: outflow obstruction from HCMP (can also cause VT), MI (more likely VT)
    Pericardial: tamponade
    Vascular: PE, PHT, aortic dissection, ruptured AAA, subclavian steal
- **Orthostatic hypotension** (~10%)
  hypovolemia/diuretics, deconditioning; vasodilat. (espec if combined w/ ⊖ chronotropes)
  autonomic neuropathy
    1° = Parkinson's, Shy-Drager, Lewy body dementia, postural orthostatic tachycardia syndrome (POTS, dysautonomia in the young)
    2° = DM, EtOH, amyloidosis, CKD (NEJM 2008;358:615)
- **Neurologic** (~10%): vertebrobasilar insufficiency (occlusion, dissection or steal), impaired perfusion to all cerebral vessels (very rare), SAH
- Remainder of cases with unknown etiology
- Misc. causes of LOC (but not syncope): seizure, TIA/stroke, migraine, hypoglycemia, hypoxia, anemia, anaphylaxis, narcolepsy, psychogenic

Workup (etiology cannot be determined in ~40% of cases)
- H&P incl. orthostatic VS have highest yield and most cost-effective (Archives 2009;169:1299)
- **History** (from Pt and witnesses if available)
  activity and posture before the incident
  precipitating factors:
    exertion → AS, HCMP, PHT
    positional Δ → orthostatic hypotension
    stressors such as sight of blood, pain, emotional distress, fatigue, prolonged standing, warm environment, N/V, cough/micturition/defecation/swallowing → vasovagal
    head turning or shaving → carotid sinus hypersensitivity
    arm exercise → subclavian steal
  prodrome: sx such as diaphoresis, nausea, blurry vision for >~5 sec suggests vasovagal; abrupt onset suggests cardiac or seizure
  associated sx: chest pain (MI), palpitations (tachycardia)
  neuro: aura prior to event, neuro sx, postictal state, bowel/bladder incontinence, & lateral tongue biting suggestive of seizure; brief convulsive activity for <10 sec may occur w/ syncope & mimic seizure, but true tonic then clonic activity is indicative of seizure
- **PMH:** prior syncope, previous cardiac or neurologic dis.; no CV disease at baseline → 5% cardiac, 25% vasovagal; CV disease → 20% cardiac, 10% vasovagal (NEJM 2002;347:878)
- **Medications that may act as precipitants**
  vasodilators: α-blockers, nitrates, ACEI/ARB, CCB, hydralazine, phenothiazines, antidep.
  diuretics; ⊖ chronotropes (eg, βB and CCB)
  proarrhythmic or QT prolonging: class IA, IC or III antiarrhythmics (see "ECG")
  psychoactive drugs: antipsychotics, TCA, barbiturates, benzodiazepines, EtOH
- **Family history:** CMP, SCD, syncope (vasovagal may have genetic component)

- **Physical exam**
  VS including _orthostatics_ (⊕ if supine → standing results in >20 mmHg ↓ SBP, >10 mmHg ↓ DBP, or >10–20 bpm ↑ HR), BP in both arms
  persistently abnormal VS concerning
  cardiac: HF (↑ JVP, displ. PMI, S₃), murmurs, LVH (S₄, LV heave), PHT (RV heave, ↑ P₂)
  vascular: ✓ for asymmetric pulses, carotid/vertebral/subclavian bruits
  carotid sinus massage to assess for carotid hypersensitivity (if no bruits and no h/o TIA or stroke); ⊕ if asystole >3 sec or ↓ SBP >50 mmHg
  neurologic exam: focal findings, evidence of tongue biting; FOBT
- **ECG** (abnormal in ~50%, but only definitively identifies cause of syncope in <10%)
  Conduction abnl: SB <40 bpm, repetitive sinus pauses >3 sec, AVB (partic. Mobitz II 2° or 3°), IVCD or BBB (partic. bifascicular block or alternating BBB) (EHJ 2009;30:2631)
  Arrhythmia: ectopy, ↑ (or ↓) QT, preexcitation (WPW), Brugada, ε wave (ACM), SVT/VT
  Ischemic changes (new or old): atrial or ventricular hypertrophy
- Place on telemetry while diagnostic workup ongoing
- Lab: glc, Hb, preg test (child-bearing age ♀), ? D-dimer, ? troponin (low yield w/o other s/s)

Life-threatening dx
- _Arrhythmia:_ VT, high-grade AVB, long sinus pauses
- _Cardiovascular structural disease:_ critical AS, HCMP, tamponade, aortic dissection, PE
- _Massive hemorrhage_ (eg, large GIB, Ao rupture, splenic rupture, ectopic preg, RP bleed)
- _Neurologic:_ SAH (headache + syncope)

High-risk features (J Emerg Med 2012;42:345)
- Advanced age (? >60 y), h/o CAD, HF/CMP, valvular or congenital heart disease, arrhythmias, or FHx SCD
- Syncope c/w cardiac cause (lack of prodrome, exertional, supine, or resultant trauma) or recurrent syncope (risk of recurrence if ≥2 prior episodes >50%)
- Complaint of chest pain or dyspnea; abnl VS or cardiac, pulmonary or neuro exam
- Abnormal ECG suggesting arrhythmia, conduction abnormality, ischemia/infarction; Pt w/ PPM/ICD (unless interrogated and found to have no arrhythmia)

Disposition
- High-risk Pts should usually be admitted w/ telemetry and further testing (qv)
- Low-risk Pts may be discharged with follow-up testing
- Obvious vasovagal syncope can be discharged

Other diagnostic studies (consider based on results of H&P and ECG)
- Ambulatory ECG monitoring: if suspect arrhythmogenic syncope
  Holter monitoring (continuous ECG 24–48 h): useful if _frequent_ events
  arrhythmia + sx (4%); asx but signif. arrhythmia (13%); sx but no arrhythmia (17%)
  Event recorder (activated by Pt to record rhythm strip): limited role, as only useful if established prodrome (because must be Pt activated)
  External intermittent loop recorders (continuously saves rhythm, ∴ can be activated _after_ an event): useful for episodes (including w/o prodrome) likely to occur w/in 1 mo
  Implantable loop recorders (inserted SC; can record up to 3 y): useful for infrequent episodes (<1/mo); recommended for recurrent syncope w/o prodrome. Appears to establish a dx (often bradycardia) more frequently (55% vs 19%) than conventional testing (external loop recorder, tilt table, etc.; Circ 2001;104:46)
- Echo: consider to r/o structural heart disease (eg, CMP [incl HCMP & ACM], valvular disease [incl AS, MS, MVP], myxoma, amyloid, PHT, ± anomalous coronaries)
- ETT: espec w/ exertional syncope; r/o ischemia- or catecholamine-induced arrhythmias
- Cardiac catheterization: consider if noninvasive tests suggest ischemia
- Electrophysiologic studies (EPS, qv): consider in high-risk Pts in whom tachy or brady etiology is strongly suspected but cannot be confirmed;
  50% abnl (inducible VT, conduction abnormalities) if heart disease, but ? significance
  3–20% abnl if abnl ECG; <1% abnl if normal heart and normal ECG (Annals 1997;127:76)
- ? Tilt table testing: utility is debated due to poor Se/Sp/reproducibility; consider only if vasovagal dx suspected but cannot be confirmed by hx
- Cardiac MRI: helpful to dx ARVC if suggestive ECG, echo (RV dysfxn) or ⊕ FHx of SCD
- Neurologic studies (cerebrovascular studies, CT, MRI, EEG): if H&P suggestive; low yield

Figure 1-10 Approach to syncope

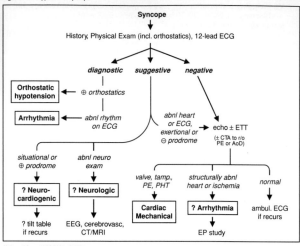

(Adapted from *JACC* 2006;47:473)

Treatment

- Arrhythmia, cardiac mechanical or neurologic syncope: treat underlying disorder
- Vasovagal syncope (*Int J Cardiol* 2013;167:1906): benefit for midodrine, SSRI
  ? 16 oz of H_2O before at-risk situations (*Circ* 2003;108:2660)
  No proven benefit w/ βB (*Circ* 2006;113:1164) or tilt training
  No benefit w/ PPM in RCT comparing active pacemaker vs pacemaker programmed in backup mode only. However, guidelines permit implant if ≥3 episodes/2y & loop recorder w/ asystole >3 sec (*Circ* 2012;125:2566).
  No data for fludrocortisone, disopyramide
- Orthostatic syncope: volume replete (eg, 500 mL PO q a.m.); if chronic → rise from supine to standing *slowly*, compressive stockings, midodrine, atomoxetine (*HTN* 2014;64:1235), fludrocortisone, high Na diet

Prognosis (*Ann Emerg Med* 1997;29:459; *NEJM* 2002;347:878)

- 22% overall recurrence rate if idiopathic, else 3% recurrence
- Cardiac syncope: 2-fold ↑ in mort., 20–40% 1-y SCD rate, median survival ~6 y
- Unexplained syncope w/ 1.3-fold ↑ in mort., but noncardiac or unexplained syncope w/ nl ECG, no h/o VT, no HF, age <45 → low recurrence rate and <5% 1-y SCD rate
- Vasovagal syncope: Pts not at increased risk for death, MI or stroke
- ✓ state driving laws and MD reporting requirements. Consider appropriateness of Pt involvement in exercise/sport, operating machinery, high-risk occupation (eg, pilot).

Procainamide (class IA = moderate Na channel blocker)

Dose	10–15 mg/kg IV over 1 h; 1–2 g bid (oral form not available in U.S.)
Uses	Converting AF & maint. SR; emergent Rx of VT or WCT of ? etiology
Side effects	↑ QT, TdP. HoTN (w/ IV use); lupus-like synd. Metab by hepatic N-acetylation. NAPA K channel blocker and renally cleared; ✓ proc & NAPA levels.

Quinidine (class IA = moderate Na channel blocker)

Dose	200–648 mg tid (slowly uptitrate); can be given IV
Uses	Prevention of VT (used mainly in refractory cases). Blocks I_{TO} (Rx VF storms in Brugada syndrome).
Side effects	↑ QT, TdP. Diarrhea often limiting. Moderate anticholinergic effects. α blockade → HoTN. Tinnitus, hemolytic anemia, thrombocytopenia.

Disopyramide (Norpace) (class IA = moderate Na channel blocker)

Dose	200–600 mg bid (slowly uptitrate)
Uses	Rx for AF in HCMP, Rx for HCMP (b/c ⊖ inotrope)
Side effects	↑ QT, TdP. Marked anticholinergic effects. ⊖ inotrope (∴ contraindic in Pts w/ ↓ EF).

Lidocaine (class IB = mild Na channel blocker)

Mech	Blocks activated & inactivated but not resting Na channels; ∴ selectively blocks ischemic arrhythmogenic tissue
Dose	100 mg IVB, subsequent 50 mg IVB prn × 2; infusion 1–4 mg/min
Uses	Emergent treatment of VT/VF
Side effects	Δ MS, slurred speech, twitching; ✓ lido levels, toxicity can manifest as seizure
Other	**Mexiletine:** IB that can be given PO (200–300 tid) to suppress VT/VF

Flecainide (Tambocor) (class IC = marked Na channel blocker)

Dose	50–150 mg bid (slowly uptitrate); 200–300 mg × 1 (pill-in-pocket)
Uses	Maintenance of SR (PAF, PSVT); acute cardioversion (test in-hosp first!) PreRx with AV nodal blocker to prevent rapid ventricular conduction.
Side effects	↑ mortality if structural heart disease (∴ contraindic if ischemic or structural heart disease). Metallic taste, negative inotropy.
Other	**Propafenone** (Rhythmol): similar indications & contrindic. Also βB. 150–300 mg tid or 225–425 bid (slowly uptitrate); 450–600 mg × 1 (pill-in-pocket).

Amiodarone (Cordarone) (class III = K channel blocker)

Mech	Primarily K channel blocker, but also Na channel blocker, βB, & CCB
Dose	IV load: 150 mg over 10 min → 1 mg/min × 6 h → 0.5 mg/min × 18 h → cont IV drip or Δ PO load for total ~10 g. PO load: 400 mg tid → total ~10 g. Maintenance: 200 (for AF) to 400 (for VT) qd. Emergent Rx of VT/VF: 300 mg IVB ± another 150 mg IVB if persists/recurs
Uses	Cardioversion AF & maintenance of SR; treatment & suppression of VT/VF
Side effects	HoTN when given IV; bradycardia. Hypo- (~10%) or hyper- (~3%, typically in iodine-defic Pts) thyroidism ↑ LFTs; pneumonitis or pulmonary fibrosis.
Other	**Dronedarone:** noniodine-containing derivative of amio w/ ↓ efficacy but better tolerability. Used for paroxysmal AF (400 mg bid). Contraindic if HF or perm AF.

Sotalol (Betapace) (class III = K channel blocker)

Mech	K+ blocker, and nonselective βB d and l isomers, respectively
Dose	Start 80 mg bid, ↑ to 120 and then up to 160 mg bid as needed.
Uses	Maintenance of SR in Pts w/ AF, prevention of VT in pts with ICD
Side effects	↑ QT (contraindic if QTc >450 msec, adjust dose to keep <500 ms). TdP. ∴ monitor in hospital for ≥3 days on maintenance dose. Renally cleared.

Ibutilide (Corvert) (class III = K channel blocker)

Dose	1 mg IV over 10 min, may repeat × 1. Mg 2 g IV routinely during infusion.
Uses	Conversion of AF
Side effects	↑ QT, TdP (~5%). Replete K & Mg before Rx. Continuous ECG monitoring (including for several hrs after last dose) and be prepared to defibrillate.
Other	**Dofetilide** (Tikosyn): maintenance of SR in Pts w/ AF. 0.5 mg bid. ↑ QT, TdP.

ELECTROPHYSIOLOGY STUDY (EPS)

Indications
- Syncope (w/ high-risk features or abnl ECG); identification of unsuspected tachyarrhythmias; distal conduction disease (not good for ruling out paroxysmal sinus node dysfunction)
- Determination of mechanism of narrow [eg, AVNRT (dual AV node physiology), AVRT (bypass tract), ectopic atrial tachycardia] and wide complex tachycardias
- Diagnosis in Pts post cardiac arrest
- Risk stratification for SCD (ie, inducibility of VT/VF) in structural heart disease

Preprocedural evaluation
- Coronary angiography to r/o signif CAD (either as cause of ischemia-induced arrhythmia and/or to fix before inducing VT)
- TEE to r/o LA clot before left atrial procedures

Commonly used catheters and measurements
- Most often electrode catheters placed via femoral vein and placed at high right atrium (HRA), His bundle (HBE) and right ventricular apex (RVA). For SVT, also have a catheter in coronary sinus (CS), coursing to left side of heart around mitral annulus.

Figure 1-11 Tracing from EPS

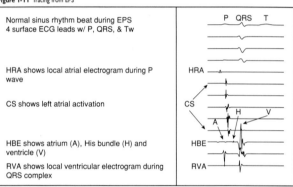

Normal sinus rhythm beat during EPS 4 surface ECG leads w/ P, QRS, & Tw	P QRS T
HRA shows local atrial electrogram during P wave	HRA
CS shows left atrial activation	CS
HBE shows atrium (A), His bundle (H) and ventricle (V)	HBE
RVA shows local ventricular electrogram during QRS complex	RVA

- His bundle electrogram allows measurement of AVN conduction (AH interval) and distal conduction system (HV interval, nl 35–55 ms):
  HV interval <35 ms: pre-excitation (WPW)
  HV interval >35 ms: conduction system disease. LBBB typically 55–65 ms, >70 ms w/ syncope needs PPM, >100 ms needs PPM
- Current driven through electrodes used to pace heart and introduce extra beats following 8-beat drive train (programmed electrical stimulation, PES) usually done at HRA and RVA
- Atrial PES can be used to reveal evidence of dual AVN pathways or accessory pathways. Can also be used to induce SVT, AF, AFL.
- Ventricular PES can be used to reveal evidence of concealed accessory pathways, assess inducibility of VT/VF (and thereby risk of SCD), particularly in ischemic heart disease.
- Drug infusions (eg, epinephrine, procainamide) can help to dx LQTS, CPVT and Brugada

Complications
- Vascular injury at site of access
- Damage to tricuspid valve
- Arrhythmias
- Cardiac chamber perforation ± tamponade
- If ablation:
  heart block ± need for PPM
  chamber perforation ± tamponade
  for AF ablation: PV stenosis, phrenic nerve injury, atrio-esophageal fistula

CARDIAC RHYTHM MANAGEMENT DEVICES

Pacemaker Code				
A, atrial; V, vent; O, none; I, inhibition; D, dual; R, rate-adaptive	**1st letter**	**2nd letter**	**3rd letter**	**4th letter**
	Chamber paced	Chamber sensed	Response to sensed beat	Program features

Common Pacing Modes	
VVI	Ventricular pacing on demand w/ single lead in RV. Sensed ventricular beat inhibits V pacing. Used in chronic AF with symptomatic bradycardia.
DDD	A & V sensing/pacing (RA & RV leads). Native A beat inhib A pacing & triggers V pacing → tracking of intrinsic atrial activity. Maintains AV synchrony, ↓ AF.
Mode Switch	In atrial tachyarrhythmia (usually atrial flutter or fibrillation), pacemaker switches from DDD to nontracking mode (like VVI) in order to prevent pacing the ventricle at the upper rate limit (max rate at which PPM will pace ventricle) in an attempt to track the rapid atrial arrhythmia
Magnet (place over generator)	Pacemaker will pace at fixed rate regardless of intrinsic activity (= VOO/DOO). ICD: no detection/shock, but pacing programming preserved. Indications: ✓ ability to capture; ✓ battery life (to which rate will be proportional; uses less energy than programmer and does not require a programmer); during surgery w/ electrocautery; hemodynamic instability due to inappropriate PPM inhib, failure to mode switch or PM-mediated tachy; inapprop ICD shocks.

Indications for Permanent Pacing *(Circ 2012;126:1784)*	
AV block	3° or type II 2° AVB a/w sx or w/ either HR <40 or asystole ≥3 sec (≥5 sec if in AF) while awake; ? asx 3° or type II 2° AVB; bifascicular or alternating left & right BBB
Sinus node	SB, pauses, chronotropic incompet a/w sx or ? if sx w/o clear assoc
Tachy-arrhythmia	Most common: AF w/ SSS, where pacing permits rate support of sinus rhythm in setting of rate controlling drugs for episodes of AF Pacing after AV junctional ablation for uncontrolled rates in AF Sustained pause-dependent VT Selected Pts w/ congenital long QT may benefit from pre-emptive pacing from their ICD
Syncope	Carotid sinus hypersensitivity with asystole >3 sec ? Neurocardiogenic syncope w/ prominent cardioinhib. response ? Syncope with bi/trifascicular block and not likely 2° to other causes

Pacing Complications (Pacemaker or ICD)		
Issue	**Manifestation**	**Description**
Failure to pace	Bradycardia	Oversensing (ie, inappropriate inhibition) due to noise from lead fracture or set screw problem, myopotentials, EMI source outside body such as electrocautery or metal detector Sensitivity too low Battery depletion
Failure to capture	Pacing impulses delivered, but no P waves or QRS evoked	Elevated pacing threshold due to lead dislodgement, local tissue reaction or injury
Failure to sense	Inapprop. pacing	Lead dislodgment or disease of local myocardium (measured electrogram from leads too small to sense) or sensing threshold too high
PM-mediated tachycardia	WCT at device upper rate	Seen w/ DDD. VA retrograde conduction; sensed by A lead → triggers V pacing → etc.
PM syndrome	Palpit, HF	Seen w/ VVI in Pts w/ intact AV conduction, due to loss of AV synchrony
SVC syndrome	Facial plethora	Thrombosis acutely or scarring a/w chronic intravascular lead(s)
Infection	Fever, ⊕ BCx	See below

Cardiac resynch therapy (CRT)/Biventricular (BiV) pacing (*Circ* 2012;126:1784)

- LBBB and standard RV apical pacing w/ resultant LBBB-like morphology causes dyssynchrony: LV septum activated before LV lateral wall. Wasted myocardial energy due to: prolonged time of contraction (sometimes continuing after AoV closure), sequential rather than simultaneous activation of papillary muscles → functional MR.
- 3-lead pacemaker (RA, RV, coronary sinus to LV lateral wall – LV lead can also be placed surgically by thoracotomy); pre-excites LV lateral wall in attempt to overcome dyssynchrony. R>S in V_1 & predominantly negative in I suggests approp LV capture. QRS width depends on degree of LV pre-excitation; can be narrower or wider than baseline.
- **Indications:** LVEF ≤35% + NYHA II–IV despite med Rx + SR + LBBB ≥150 (? ≥120) ms; mortality benefit only if LBBB (regardless of QRS width) (*NEJM* 2014;370:1694)
  can also consider in AF, but rate control or AVN ablation necessary to allow ventricular capture, as the greater proportion of time paced, the greater the CRT effect;
  ? NYHA I w/ LVEF ≤30% + LBBB ≥150 ms;
  ? EF ≤50% w/ AVB + indic for PPM (*NEJM* 2013;368:1585)
- **Benefits**
  acutely: simultaneous contraction of LV walls and reduction in MR
  after 3–6 mo: improvement in one NYHA class in 2/3 of Pts; some "super-responders" will normalize EF
  clinically: ↓ HF sx, ↓ HF hosp., ↑ survival (*NEJM* 2005;352:1539; 2010;363:2385)
  ineffective when LV lead location poor or LV scarring prevents pacing and/or improvements in wall motion

Implantable cardiac defibrillator (ICD) (*NEJM* 2003;349:1836; *JACC* 2009;54:747)

- RV lead: pacing and sensing like pacemaker lead, coils plus outside housing of ICD can participate in shocking circuit (± antitachycardia pacing [ATP] = burst pacing faster than VT rate to stop VT w/o painful shocks); ± RA lead for dual chamber pacing
- Uninterrupted warfarin at time of ICD (or PPM) placement ↓ risk of pocket hematoma vs bridging with UFH (*NEJM* 2013;368:2084)
- Subcutaneous ICD contains only shocking function (no ATP, no pacing) implanted in the left parasternal area with pulse generator in left lateral thoracic area. Reasonable for those with poor central access and those w/o pacing requirement (*Circ* 2013;127:854).
- Wearable defibrillator vest can act as a "bridge" for Pts who cannot have an implanted defibrillator for weeks to a few months due to infection or other issue. Not yet demonstrated benefit as a bridge for those who do not yet meet guidelines for ICD (eg, early post MI or new NICMP) (*JACC* 2013;62:2000). Data do not support home AED for these Pts either (*NEJM* 2018;358:1793).
- **Pt selection** (*NEJM* 2004;350:2151 & 351:2481; 2005;352:225; 2009;361:1427; *Circ* 2012;126:1784)
  2° prevention: survivors of VF arrest, unstable VT w/o reversible cause (*NEJM* 1997;337:1576); structural heart disease & spontaneous sustained VT (even if asx)
  1° prevention:
  LVEF ≤30% & post-MI or LVEF ≤35% & NYHA II-III or LVEF ≤40% & inducible VT/VF
  wait ≥40 d if post-MI, >9 mo after dx of NICM, or if presumed reversible;
  however, consider ICD if hemodyn signif VT/VF w/in window (& >48 h after AMI) (*Circ* 2014;130:94)
  consider for HCM, ARVC, Brugada, sarcoid, LQTS, Chagas or congenital heart disease if risk factors for SCD
  life expectancy must be >1 y
- **Benefits:** ↓ mortality from SCD c/w antiarrhythmics or placebo
- **Risks:** inapprop shock in ~15–20% at 3 y (most commonly due to misclassified SVT); lead fracture
- ICD discharge: ✓ device to see if approp; r/o ischemia, other proximate cause; if recurrent VT, ? drug Rx (eg, amio + βB; *JAMA* 2006;295:165) or VT ablation (*NEJM* 2007;357:2657); ablation at time of ICD ↓ risk of VT by 40% (*Lancet* 2010;375:31)
- Telemonitoring may improve outcomes (*Lancet* 2014;384:583)

Device infection (*Circ* 2010;121:458; *JAMA* 2012;307:1727; *NEJM* 2012;367:842)

- Presents with one or more of the following: pocket infection (warmth, erythema, tenderness), fever, bacteremia and/or sepsis
- Incidence ~2% over 5 y; if S. aureus bacteremia, infxn in ≥35%
- More common a complication of generator change
- TTE/TEE used to help visualize complic. (eg, vegetation), but even ⊖ TEE does not r/o
- Treatment: abx and removal of system if evidence of pocket infection or GPC bacteremia (*Heart Rhythm* 2009;7:1085)
- Prophylaxis: no recommendation for routine abx prior to invasive procedure

Drug	Class	Dose	
		per kg	average
Pressors, Inotropes and Chronotropes			
Phenylephrine	α₁	10–300 mcg/min	
Norepinephrine	α₁ > β₁	1–40 mcg/min	
Vasopressin	V₁	0.01–0.1 U/min (usually <0.04)	
Epinephrine	α₁, α₂, β₁, β₂	2–20 mcg/min	
Isoproterenol	β₁, β₂	0.1–10 mcg/min	
Dopamine	D	0.5–2 mcg/kg/min	50–200 mcg/min
	β, D	2–10 mcg/kg/min	200–500 mcg/min
	α, β, D	>10 mcg/kg/min	500–1000 mcg/min
Dobutamine	β₁ > β₂	2–20 mcg/kg/min	50–1000 mcg/min
Milrinone	PDE	± 50 mcg/kg over 10 min then 0.25–0.75 mcg/kg/min	3–4 mg over 10 min then 20–50 mcg/min
Vasodilators			
Nitroglycerin	NO	10–1000 mcg/min	
Nitroprusside	NO	0.25–10 mcg/kg/min	10–800 mcg/min
Labetalol	α₁, β₁ and β₂ blocker	20–80 mg q10min or 10–120 mg/h	
Fenoldopam	D	0.1–1.6 mcg/kg/min	10–120 mg/h
Clevidipine	CCB	1–16 mg/h	
Epoprostenol	vasodilator	2–20 ng/kg/min	
Antiarrhythmics			
Amiodarone	K et al. (Class III)	150 mg over 10 min, then 1 mg/min × 6 h, then 0.5 mg/min × 18 h	
Lidocaine	Na channel (Class IB)	1–1.5 mg/kg then 1–4 mg/min	100 mg then 1–4 mg/min
Procainamide	Na channel (Class IA)	17 mg/kg over 60 min then 1–4 mg/min	1 g over 60 min then 1–4 mg/min
Ibutilide	K channel (Class III)	1 mg over 10 min, may repeat × 1	
Propranolol	β blocker	0.5–1 mg q5min then 1–10 mg/h	
Esmolol	β₁ > β₂ blocker	500 mcg/kg then 50–200 mcg/kg/min	20–40 mg over 1 min then 2–20 mg/min
Verapamil	CCB	2.5–5 mg over 1–2′, repeat 5–10 mg in 15–30′ prn 5–20 mg/h	
Diltiazem	CCB	0.25 mg/kg over 2 min reload 0.35 mg/kg × 1 prn then 5–15 mg/h	20 mg over 2 min reload 25 mg × 1 prn then 5–15 mg/h
Adenosine	purinergic	6-mg rapid push; if no response: 12 mg → 12–18 mg	
Sedation			
Morphine	opioid	1–30 (in theory, unlimited) mg/h	
Fentanyl	opioid	50–100 mcg then 50–800 (? unlimited) mcg/h	
Propofol	anesthetic	1–3 mg/kg then 0.3–5 mg/kg/h	50–200 mg then 20–400 mg/h
Dexmedetomidine	α₂ agonist	1 mcg/kg over 10 min → 0.2–0.7 mcg/kg/h	
Diazepam	BDZ	1–5 mg q1–2h then q6h prn	
Midazolam	BDZ	0.5–2 mg q5min prn; 0.02–0.1 mg/kg/h or 1–10 mg/h	
Lorazepam	BDZ	0.01–0.1 mg/kg/h	
Naloxone	opioid antag.	0.4–2 mg q2–3min to total of 10 mg	
Flumazenil	BDZ antag.	0.2 mg over 30 sec then 0.3 mg over 30 sec prn may repeat 0.5 mg over 30 sec to total of 3 mg	

Drug	Class	Dose	
		per kg	average
Miscellaneous			
Aminophylline	PDE	5.5 mg/kg over 20 min then 0.5–1 mg/kg/h	250–500 mg then 10–80 mg/h
Octreotide	somatostatin analog	50 mcg then 50 mcg/h	
Mannitol	osmole	1.5–2 g/kg over 30–60 min repeat q6–12h to keep osm 310–320	

TREATMENT OF HYPOTENSION/SHOCK

Figure Appendix-1 ACLS pulmonary edema, hypotension or shock algorithm

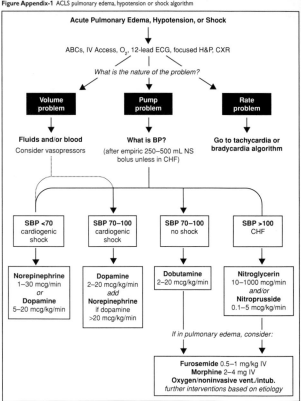

(Adapted from ACLS 2005 Guidelines)

CARDIOLOGY

Hemodynamic parameters	Normal value
Mean arterial pressure (MAP) $= \dfrac{SBP + (DBP \times 2)}{3}$	70–100 mmHg
Heart rate (HR)	60–100 bpm
Right atrial pressure (RA)	≤6 mmHg
Right ventricular (RV)	systolic 15–30 mmHg diastolic 1–8 mmHg
Pulmonary artery (PA)	systolic 15–30 mmHg mean 9–18 mmHg diastolic 6–12 mmHg
Pulmonary capillary wedge pressure (PCWP)	≤12 mmHg
Cardiac output (CO)	4–8 L/min
Cardiac index (CI) $= \dfrac{CO}{BSA}$	2.6–4.2 L/min/m^2
Stroke volume (SV) $= \dfrac{CO}{HR}$	60–120 mL/contraction
Stroke volume index (SVI) $= \dfrac{CI}{HR}$	40–50 mL/contraction/m^2
Systemic vascular resistance (SVR) $= \dfrac{MAP - mean\,RA}{CO} \times 80$	800–1200 dynes × sec/cm^5
Pulmonary vascular resistance (PVR) $= \dfrac{mean\,PA - mean\,PCWP}{CO} \times 80$	120–250 dynes × sec/cm^5

"Rule of 6s" for PAC: RA ≤6, RV ≤30/6, PA ≤30/12, WP ≤12. Nb 1 mmHg = 1.36 cm water or blood.

Fick cardiac output
Oxygen consumption (L/min) = CO (L/min) × arteriovenous (AV) oxygen difference
CO = oxygen consumption/AV oxygen difference
Oxygen consumption must be measured (can estimate w/ 125 mL/min/m^2 but inaccurate)
AV oxygen difference = Hb (g/dL) × 10 (dL/L) × 1.36 (mL O_2/g of Hb) × ($S_aO_2 - S_{MV}O_2$)
   S_aO_2 is measured in any arterial sample (usually 93–98%)
   $S_{MV}O_2$ (mixed venous O_2) is measured in RA, RV or PA (assuming no shunt) (nl ~75%)

∴ **Cardiac output** (L/min) $= \dfrac{Oxygen\ consumption}{Hb\ (g/dL) \times 13.6\ (S_aO_2 - S_{MV}O_2)}$

Shunts
$Q_p = \dfrac{Oxygen\ consumption}{Pulm.\ vein\ O_2\ sat - Pulm.\ artery\ O_2\ sat}$ (if no R → L shunt, PV O_2 sat ≈ S_aO_2)

$Q_s = \dfrac{Oxygen\ consumption}{S_aO_2 - mixed\ venous\ O_2\ sat}$ (MVO_2 drawn proximal to potential L → R shunt)

$\dfrac{Q_p}{Q_s} = \dfrac{S_aO_2 - MV\,O_2\ sat}{PV\,O_2\ sat - PA\,O_2\ sat} \approx \dfrac{S_aO_2 - MV\,O_2\ sat}{S_aO_2 - PA\,O_2\ sat}$ (if only L → R and no R → L shunt)

Valve equations
Simplified Bernoulli: Pressure gradient (ΔP) = 4 × v^2 (where v = peak flow velocity)
Continuity (conservation of flow): Area$_1$ × Velocity$_1$ = A$_2$ × V$_2$ (where 1 & 2 different points)

   or AVA (unknown) = A$_{LV\ outflow\ tract}$ × $\left(\dfrac{V_{LVOT}}{V_{AoV}}\right)$ (all of which can be measured on echo)

Gorlin equation: Valve area $= \dfrac{CO/(DEP\ or\ SEP) \times HR}{44.3 \times constant \times \sqrt{\Delta P}}$ (constant = 1 for AS, 0.85 for MS)

Hakki equation: Valve area $\approx \dfrac{CO}{\sqrt{\Delta P}}$

Heparin for Thromboembolism	
80 U/kg bolus	
18 U/kg/h	
PTT	**Adjustment**
<40	bolus 5000 U, ↑ rate 300 U/h
40–49	bolus 3000 U, ↑ rate 200 U/h
50–59	↑ rate 150 U/h
60–85	no Δ
86–95	↓ rate 100 U/h
96–120	hold 30 min, ↓ rate 100 U/h
>120	hold 60 min, ↓ rate 150 U/h

(Modified from Chest 2008;133:141S)

Heparin for ACS	
60 U/kg bolus (max 4000 U)	
12 U/kg/h (max 1000 U/h)	
PTT	**Adjustment**
<40	bolus 3000 U, ↑ rate 100 U/h
40–49	↑ rate 100 U/h
50–75	no Δ
76–85	↓ rate 100 U/h
86–100	hold 30 min, ↓ rate 100 U/h
>100	hold 60 min, ↓ rate 200 U/h

(Modified from Circ 2007;116:e148 & Chest 2008;133:670)

✓ PTT q6h after every Δ ($t_{1/2}$ of heparin ~90 min) and then qd or bid once PTT is therapeutic
✓ CBC qd (to ensure Hct and plt counts are stable)

Warfarin Loading Nomogram					
Day	**INR**				
	<1.5	**1.5–1.9**	**2–2.5**	**2.6–3**	**>3**
1–3	5 mg (7.5 mg if > 80 kg)		2.5–5 mg	0–2.5 mg	0 mg
4–5	10 mg	5–10 mg	0–5 mg		0–2.5 mg
6	Dose based on requirements over preceding 5 d				

(Annals 1997;126:133; Archives 1999;159:46) or, go to www.warfarindosing.org

Warfarin-heparin overlap therapy
- Indications: when failure to anticoagulate carries ↑ risk of morbidity or mortality (eg, DVT/PE, intracardiac thrombus)
- Rationale: (1) Half-life of factor VII (3–6 h) is shorter than half-life of factor II (60–72 h);
  ∴ warfarin can elevate PT *before achieving a true antithrombotic state*
  (2) Protein C also has half-life less than that of factor II;
  ∴ theoretical concern of *hypercoagulable state* before antithrombotic state
- Method: (1) Therapeutic PTT is achieved using heparin
  (2) Warfarin therapy is initiated
  (3) Heparin continued until INR therapeutic for ≥2 d and ≥4–5 d of warfarin (roughly corresponds to ~2 half-lives of factor II or a reduction to ~25%)

Common Warfarin-Drug Interactions	
Drugs that ↑ PT	**Drugs that ↓ PT**
Amiodarone	Antimicrobials: rifampin
Antimicrobials: erythromycin, ? clarithro, ciprofloxacin, MNZ, sulfonamides	CNS: barbiturates, carbamazepine, phenytoin (initial transient ↑ PT)
Antifungals: azoles	Cholestyramine
Acetaminophen, cimetidine, levothyroxine	

ABBREVIATIONS

AAA	abdominal aortic aneurysm	bx	biopsy
AAD	antiarrhythmic drug	c/s	consult
ABE	acute bacterial endocarditis	c/w	compared with
ABI	ankle-brachial index		consistent with
abnl	abnormal	CABG	coronary artery bypass grafting
abx	antibiotics		
ACE	angiotensin converting enzyme	CAC	coronary artery calcium
		CAD	coronary artery disease
ACEI	ACE inhibitor	CBC	complete blood count
ACL	anticardiolipin antibody	CCB	calcium channel blocker
ACLS	advanced cardiac life support	CCS	Canadian Cardiovascular Society
ACM	arrhythmogenic cardiomyopathy		
ACS	acute coronary syndrome	CCTA	coronary CT angiography
ADL	activities of daily living	CEA	carotid endarterectomy
AED	automated external defib.	CHB	complete heart block
AF	atrial fibrillation	CHD	congenital heart disease
AFB	acid-fast bacilli	CHF	congestive heart failure
AFL	atrial flutter	CI	cardiac index
AI	aortic insufficiency	CIAKI	contrast-induced AKI
AIVR	accelerated idioventric. rhythm	CIED	cardiac implantable electronic device
AKI	acute kidney injury	CK	creatine kinase
AL	amyloidosis	CKD	chronic kidney disease
ALT	alanine aminotransferase	CMP	cardiomyopathy
AMI	acute myocardial infarction	CMV	cytomegalovirus
	anterior myocardial infarction	CNS	central nervous system
ANA	antinuclear antibody	CO	cardiac output
APB	atrial premature beat	COPD	chronic obstructive pulmonary disease
AoD	aortic dissection		
AoV	aortic valve	COX	cyclo-oxygenase
aPTT	activated PTT	CP	chest pain
AR	aortic regurgitation	Cr	creatinine
ARB	angiotensin receptor blocker	Cr Cl	creatinine clearance
ARDS	acute resp. distress syndrome	CRP	C-reactive protein
ARNi	angiotensin receptor neprilysin inhibitor	CRT	cardiac resynchronization therapy
ARVC	arrhythmogenic RV CMP	CS	coronary sinus
AS	aortic stenosis	CsA	cyclosporine A
ASA	aspirin	CT	computed tomogram
ASD	atrial septal defect	CTA	CT angiogram
asx	asymptomatic	CTD	connective tissue disease
AT	atrial tachycardia	CTEPH	chronic thromboembolic pulmonary HTN
ATII	angiotensin II		
ATP	antitachycardia pacing	CV	cardiovascular
AV	atrioventricular	CVA	cerebrovascular accident
AVA	aortic valve area	CVD	cerebrovascular disease
AVB	atrioventricular block		collagen vascular disease
AVM	arteriovenous malformation	CVP	central venous pressure
AVN	AV node	CW	chest wall
AVNRT	AVN reentrant tachycardia	CXR	chest radiograph
AVR	aortic valve replacement		
AVRT	AV reciprocating tachycardia	d	day
a/w	associated with	D	death
AZA	azathioprine	∆MS	change in mental status
		DAPT	dual antiplatelet therapy
b/c	because	DBP	diastolic blood pressure
βB	beta-blocker	d/c	discharge
BaV	balloon AoV valvotomy		discontinue
BBB	bundle branch block	DCCV	direct current cardioversion
BCx	blood culture	DCM(P)	dilated cardiomyopathy
BiV	biventricular	Ddx	differential diagnosis
BMI	body mass index	DES	drug-eluting stent
BMS	bare metal stent	DM	dermatomyositis
BNP	B-type natriuretic peptide		diabetes mellitus
BP	blood pressure	DOE	dyspnea on exertion
BS	breath sounds	DSE	dobutamine stress echo
BSA	body surface area	DVT	deep vein thrombosis
BUN	blood urea nitrogen	dx	diagnosis

EAD	extreme axis deviation	**INH**	isoniazid
EBV	Epstein-Barr virus	**INR**	international normalized ratio
ECG	electrocardiogram	**IVB**	intravenous bolus
ECMO	extracorporeal membrane oxygenation	**IVC**	inferior vena cava
		IVCD	interventricular conduction delay
ED	emergency department		
EDP	end-diastolic pressure	**IVF**	intravenous fluids
EDV	end-diastolic volume	**IVIg**	intravenous immunoglobulin
EF	ejection fraction		
EGD	esophagogastroduodenoscopy	**JVP**	jugular venous pulse
EP	electrophysiology		
EPS	electrophysiology study	**LA**	left atrium
ERO	effective regurgitant orifice	**LAA**	left atrial abnormality
ESP	end-systolic pressure		left atrial appendage
ESR	erythrocyte sedimentation rate	**LAD**	left anterior descending cor. art.
			left axis deviation
ESRD	end-stage renal disease	**LAE**	left atrial enlargement
ESV	end-systolic volume	**LAFB**	left anterior fascicular block
EtOH	alcohol	**LAP**	left atrial pressure
ETT	exercise tolerance test	**LBBB**	left bundle branch block
EVAR	endovascular aneurysm repair	**LCA**	left coronary artery
		LCx	left circumflex cor. art.
FFP	fresh frozen plasma	**LD**	loading dose
FFR	fractional flow reserve	**LDH**	lactate dehydrogenase
FH	familial hypercholesterolemia	**LDL**	low-density lipoprotein
FHx	family history	**LFTs**	liver function tests
FMD	fibromuscular dysplasia	**LIMA**	left internal mammary artery
FOBT	fecal occult blood testing	**LLSB**	lower left sternal border
		LM	left main coronary artery
GCA	giant cell arteritis	**LMWH**	low-molecular-weight heparin
GCM	giant cell myocarditis	**LOC**	loss of consciousness
GFR	glomerular filtration rate	**LOS**	length of stay
GIB	gastrointestinal bleed	**LPFB**	left posterior fascicular block
glc	glucose	**LR**	likelihood ratio
GPC	gram-positive cocci	**LQTS**	long QT syndrome
GPI	glycoprotein IIb/IIIa inhibitor	**LUSB**	left upper sternal border
GRA	glucocorticoid-remediable aldosteronism	**LV**	left ventricle
		LVAD	LV assist device
h	hour	**LVEDP**	LV end-diastolic pressure
HA	headache	**LVEDV**	LV end-diastolic volume
HCM(P)	hypertrophic cardiomyopathy	**LVESD**	LV end-systolic diameter
Hct	hematocrit	**LVH**	left ventricular hypertrophy
HCV	hepatitis C virus	**LVOT**	left ventricular outflow tract
HD	hemodialysis	**LVSD**	LV systolic dimension
HDL	high-density lipoprotein		
HF	heart failure	**mAb**	monoclonal antibody
HFpEF	HF with preserved EF	**MAC**	mitral annular calcification
HFrEF	HF with reduced EF	**MACE**	major adverse CV event
HIT	heparin-induced thrombocytopenia	**MAO**	monoamine oxidase
		MAP	mean arterial pressure
HK	hypokinesis	**MAT**	multifocal atrial tachycardia
h/o	history of	**MCS**	mechanical circulatory support
HOB	head of bed	**METs**	metabolic equivalent of task
HoTN	hypotension	**MGUS**	monoclonal gammopathy of uncertain significance
HR	heart rate		
HTN	hypertension	**MI**	myocardial infarction
hx	history	**min**	minute
		min.	minimal
I	iodine	**MM**	multiple myeloma
IABP	intra-aortic balloon pump	**MMVT**	monomorphic ventricular tachycardia
IC	intracoronary		
ICD	implantable cardiac defibrillator	**mo**	month
		mod.	moderate
ICH	intracranial hemorrhage	**MR**	magnetic resonance
ICP	intracranial pressure		mitral regurgitation
IDL	intermediate-density lipoprotein	**MRA**	magnetic resonance angiography
		MRI	magnetic resonance imaging
IE	infective endocarditis	**MS**	mitral stenosis
IHD	ischemic heart disease		mental status
IMI	inferior myocardial infarction	**MTb**	*Mycobacterium tuberculosis*

MTX	methotrexate		PNA	pneumonia
MV	mitral valve		PND	paroxysmal nocturnal dyspnea
MVA	mitral valve area		PO	oral intake
MVP	mitral valve prolapse		POBA	plain old balloon angioplasty
MVR	mitral valve replacement		POTS	postural orthostatic tachycardia syndrome
MWD	minute walking distance		PPH	primary pulmonary HTN
			PPI	proton pump inhibitors
N/V	nausea and/or vomiting		PPM	permanent pacemaker
NAC	N-acetylcysteine		PPV	positive predictive value
NICM(P)	nonischemic cardiomyopathy		Ppx	prophylaxis
nl	normal		PR	PR segment on ECG
NO	nitric oxide			pulmonary regurgitation
NPJT	nonparoxysmal junctional tachycardia		PRBCs	packed red blood cells
NPO	nothing by mouth		PRWP	poor R wave progression
NPV	negative predictive value		PS	pressure support
NS	normal saline			pulmonic stenosis
NSAID	nonsteroidal anti-inflam. drug		PSVT	paroxysmal supravent. tachycardia
NSTE	non ST-segment elevation		Pt	patient
NSTEMI	non ST-segment elevation MI		PT	posterior tibialis
NSVT	nonsustained ventricular tachycardia			prothrombin time
NTG	nitroglycerin		PTA	perc. transluminal angioplasty
NVE	native valve endocarditis		PTT	partial thromboplastin time
NYHA	New York Heart Association		PTX	pneumothorax
NVAF	non-valvular AF		PUD	peptic ulcer disease
			PV	portal vein
OCP	oral contraceptive pill		PVC	premature ventricular contraction
O/D	overdose		PVD	peripheral vasc. disease
OM	obtuse marginal cor. art.		PVR	pulmonary vascular resistance
OMT	optimal medical therapy		p/w	presents with
OSA	obstructive sleep apnea			
			QoL	quality of life
PA	pulmonary artery		Qw	Q wave
PAC	pulmonary artery catheter			
PAD	peripheral artery disease		RA	refractory anemia
PAF	paroxysmal atrial fibrillation			rheumatoid arthritis
PAN	polyarteritis nodosa			right atrium
PAP	PA pressure		RAA	renin-angiotensin-aldosterone
PASP	PA systolic pressure			right atrial abnormality
PAV	percutaneous aortic valvuloplasty			right atrial appendage
pb	problem		RAD	right axis deviation
PBC	primary biliary cirrhosis		RAE	right atrial enlargement
PCC	prothrombin complex concentrate		RAP	right atrial pressure
			RAS	renal artery stenosis
PCI	percutaneous coronary intervention		RBBB	right bundle branch block
PCKD	polycystic kidney disease		RCA	right coronary artery
PCWP	pulmonary capillary wedge pressure		RCC	renal cell carcinoma
PDA	patent ductus arteriosus		RCM(P)	restrictive cardiomyopathy
	post. descending cor. art.		RCT	randomized controlled trial
PE	pulmonary embolism		RF	risk factor
PEA	pulseless electrical activity		RFA	radio frequency ablation
PEEP	positive end-expiratory pressure		RHD	rheumatic heart disease
			r/i	rule in
PET	positron emission tomography		r/o	rule out
			RR	respiratory rate
PEx	physical exam		RUQ	right upper quadrant
PFO	patent foramen ovale		RUSB	right upper sternal border
PFT	pulmonary function test		RV	right ventricle
PHT	pulmonary hypertension		RVAD	RV assist device
plt	platelet		RVH	RV hypertrophy
PM	polymyositis		RVOT	RV outflow tract
PMHx	past medical history		RVSP	RV systolic pressure
PMI	point of maximal impulse		Rx	therapy
PMV	percutaneous mitral valvuloplasty			
			SA	sinoatrial
PMVT	polymorphic ventricular tachycardia		SAH	subarachnoid hemorrhage
			SAM	systolic anterior motion

SB	sinus bradycardia	**TPG**	transpulmonary gradient
SBE	subacute bacterial endocarditis	**TR**	tricuspid regurgitation
SBP	systolic blood pressure	**TRS**	TIMI risk score
SC	subcutaneous	**TS**	tricuspid stenosis
SCA	sudden cardiac arrest	**TTE**	transthoracic echo
SCD	sudden cardiac death	**TV**	tricuspid valve
s/e	side effect	**Tw**	T wave
Se	sensitivity	**TWF**	T-wave flattening
sec	second	**TWI**	T-wave inversion
sev.	severe	**Tx**	transplant
SIHD	stable ischemic heart disease	**TZD**	thiazolidinediones
SK	streptokinase		
SLE	systemic lupus erythematosus	**U/S**	ultrasound
SOB	shortness of breath	**UA**	unstable angina
s/p	status post		uric acid
Sp	specificity	**UFH**	unfractionated heparin
SPEP	serum protein	**ULN**	upper limit of normal
	electrophoresis	**UOP**	urine output
SR	sinus rhythm	**UPEP**	urine protein electrophoresis
s/s	signs and symptoms	**UR**	urgent revascularization
SSRI	selective serotonin reuptake		
	inhibitor	**V/Q**	ventilation-perfusion
SSS	sick sinus syndrome	**VAD**	ventricular assist device
ST	sinus tachycardia	**VD**	vessel disease
STD	ST-segment depression	**VF**	ventricular fibrillation
STE	ST-segment elevation	**VLDL**	very-low-density lipoproteins
STEMI	ST-segment elevation MI	**VOD**	veno-occlusive disease
SV	stroke volume	**VS**	vital signs
SVC	superior vena cava	**VSD**	ventricular septal defect
SVG	saphenous vein graft	**VT**	ventricular tachycardia
SVR	systemic vascular resistance	**VTE**	venous thromboembolus
SVT	supraventricular tachycardia	**vWD**	von Willebrand's disease
sx	symptom(s) or symptomatic	**vWF**	von Willebrand's factor
		VZV	varicella zoster virus
TAVR	transcatheter aortic valve		
	replacement	**w/**	with
TB	tuberculosis	**WCT**	wide-complex tachycardia
TC	total cholesterol	**wk**	week
TCA	tricyclic antidepressant	**WM**	Waldenström's
TdP	torsades de pointes		macroglobulinemia
TEE	transesophageal echo	**WMA**	wall motion abnormality
TFTs	thyroid function tests	**WPW**	Wolff-Parkinson-White
TG	triglycerides		syndrome
TGA	transposition of the great	**w/u**	workup
	arteries		
TIA	transient ischemic attack	**XRT**	radiation therapy
Tn	troponin		
TP	total protein	**y**	year

INDEX

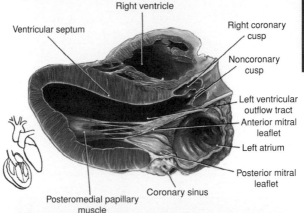

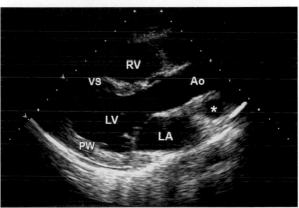

1 Parasternal long-axis view allows visualization of the right ventricle (RV), ventricular septum (VS), posterior wall (PW) aortic valve cusps, left ventricle (LV), mitral valve, left atrium (LA), and ascending thoracic aorta (Ao). *Pulmonary artery.
(Top: From *Mayo Clinic Proceedings.* [Tajik AJ, Seward JB, Hagler DJ, et al. Two-dimensional real-time ultrasonic imaging of the heart and great vessels: Technique, image orientation, structure identification, and validation. *Mayo Clinic Proceedings,* 1978;53:271–303], with permission. Bottom: From Oh JK, Seward JB, Tajik AJ. *The Echo Manual,* 3rd ed. Philadelphia: Lippincott Williams & Wilkins, 2006. By permission of Mayo Foundation for Medical Education and Research. All rights reserved.)

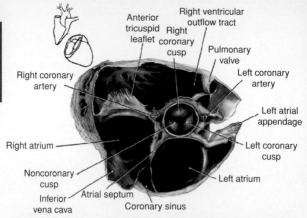

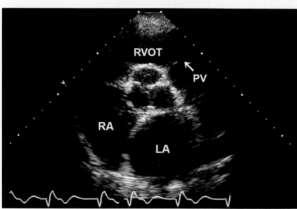

2 Parasternal short-axis view at the level of the aorta: LA, left atrium; PV, pulmonary valve; RA, right atrium; RVOT, right ventricular outflow tract. (Top: From *Mayo Clinic Proceedings.* [Tajik AJ, Seward JB, Hagler DJ, et al. Two-dimensional real-time ultrasonic imaging of the heart and great vessels: Technique, image orientation, structure identification, and validation. *Mayo Clinic Proceedings,* 1978;53:271–303], with permission. Bottom: From Oh JK, Seward JB, Tajik AJ. *The Echo Manual,* 3rd ed. Philadelphia: Lippincott Williams & Wilkins, 2006. By permission of Mayo Foundation for Medical Education and Research. All rights reserved.)

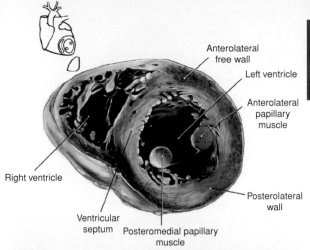

Anterolateral
free wall

Left ventricle

Anterolateral
papillary
muscle

Right ventricle

Posterolateral
wall

Ventricular
septum

Posteromedial papillary
muscle

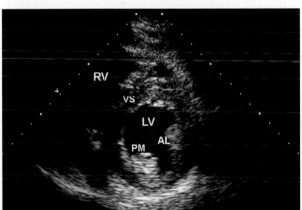

3 Parasternal short-axis view at the level of the papillary muscles: AL, anterolateral papillary muscle; PM, posteromedial papillary muscle; RV, right ventricle; VS, ventricular septum; LV, left ventricle. (Top: From *Mayo Clinic Proceedings.* [Tajik AJ, Seward JB, Hagler DJ, et al. Two-dimensional real-time ultrasonic imaging of the heart and great vessels: Technique, image orientation, structure identification, and validation. *Mayo Clinic Proceedings,* 1978;53:271–303], with permission. Bottom: From Oh JK, Seward JB, Tajik AJ. *The Echo Manual,* 3rd ed. Philadelphia: Lippincott Williams & Wilkins, 2006. By permission of Mayo Foundation for Medical Education and Research. All rights reserved.)

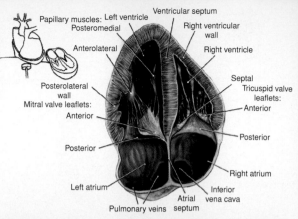

Papillary muscles: Left ventricle
Posteromedial
Ventricular septum
Right ventricular wall
Anterolateral
Right ventricle
Posterolateral wall
Mitral valve leaflets:
Anterior
Septal
Tricuspid valve leaflets:
Anterior
Posterior
Posterior
Right atrium
Left atrium
Inferior vena cava
Pulmonary veins
Atrial septum

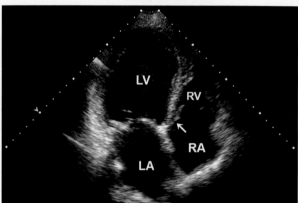

4 Apical four-chamber view: Note that at some institutions the image is reversed so that the left side of the heart appears on the right side of the screen. LA, left atrium; LV, left ventricle; RA, right atrium; RV, right ventricle. (Top: From *Mayo Clinic Proceedings.* [Tajik AJ, Seward JB, Hagler DJ, et al. Two-dimensional real-time ultrasonic imaging of the heart and great vessels: Technique, image orientation, structure identification, and validation. *Mayo Clinic Proceedings*, 1978;53:271–303], with permission. Bottom: From Oh JK, Seward JB, Tajik AJ. *The Echo Manual*, 3rd ed. Philadelphia: Lippincott Williams & Wilkins, 2006. By permission of Mayo Foundation for Medical Education and Research. All rights reserved.)

Nuclear Imaging

Images during stress are on top, and the corresponding images at rest are immediately below.

Perfusion defects that appear only during stress imaging suggest reversible myocardial ischemia, whereas perfusion defects that appear on both stress and rest images suggest irreversible scar (or artifact).

In this example, the patient has a large area of severe ischemia involving the anterior, septal, and lateral walls, from the base to the apex. There is also transient ischemic dilation of the LV cavity. These findings are consistent with severe stenosis of the proximal LAD or the left main coronary artery.

Short axis images going from the apex to the base (stress images are 1st and 3rd rows, rest images 2nd and 4th rows):

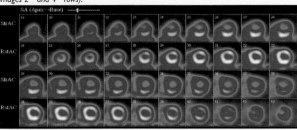

Horizontal long axis images going from the inferior to the superior surface:

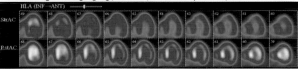

Vertical long axis images going from the inferior to the superior surface:

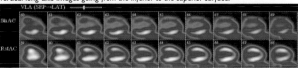

(Images from Jaber WA, Cerqueira MD. *Nuclear Cardiology Review*. Philadelphia: Lippincott Williams & Wilkins, 2013.)

Coronary Angiography

Coronary arteries are usually imaged in orthogonal planes, involving both right anterior oblique or **RAO views** (where one is looking at the "side" of the heart, with the spine of the left-hand side of the image, the atria on the left-hand side of the image, and the ventricular apex on the right-hand side) and left anterior oblique or **LAO views** (where one is looking more down the "barrel" of the heart, with the spine on the right-hand side of the image, the atria in the background, and the apex in the foreground), and **cranial angulation** (where one can see the diaphragm; often better for visualizing the LAD) and **caudal angulation** (where one cannot see the diaphragm; often better for visualizing the LCx).

Model of the coronary arteries (both left and right depicted simultaneously) in RAO and LAO views. (From Moscucci M. *Grossman & Baim's Cardiac Catheterization, Angiography, and Intervention*, 8th ed. Philadelphia: Lippincott Williams & Wilkins, 2014.)

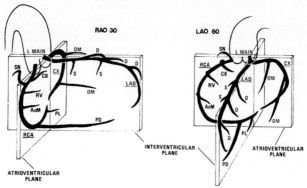

Illustrations of selective angiograms of the left and right coronary arteries. (From Grossman WG. *Cardiac Catheterization and Angiography*, 4th ed. Philadelphia: Lea & Febiger, 1991, with permission.)

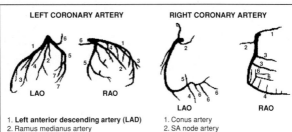

LEFT CORONARY ARTERY	RIGHT CORONARY ARTERY
1. **Left anterior descending artery (LAD)**	1. Conus artery
2. Ramus medianus artery	2. SA node artery
3. Diagonal branches	3. Acute marginal branches
4. Septal branches	4. Posterior descending artery (PDA)
5. **Left circumflex artery (LCx)**	5. AV node artery
6. Left atrial circumflex artery	6. Posterior left ventricular artery (PLV)
7. Obtuse marginal branches	

ACLS ALGORITHMS

Figure ACLS-1 ACLS Tachycardia Algorithm

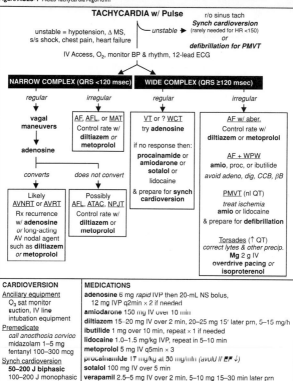

TACHYCARDIA w/ Pulse

r/o sinus tach

unstable = hypotension, Δ MS,
s/s shock, chest pain, heart failure

unstable → *Synch cardioversion*
(rarely needed for HR <150)
or
defibrillation for PMVT

IV Access, O₂, monitor BP & rhythm, 12-lead ECG

NARROW COMPLEX (QRS <120 msec) | **WIDE COMPLEX (QRS ≥120 msec)**

regular — **vagal maneuvers** → **adenosine**

converts → Likely **AVNRT or AVRT** Rx recurrence w/ **adenosine** or long-acting AV nodal agent such as **diltiazem** or **metoprolol**

does not convert → Possibly **AFL, ATAC, NPJT** Control rate w/ **diltiazem** or **metoprolol**

irregular — **AF, AFL, or MAT** Control rate w/ **diltiazem** or **metoprolol**

regular — **VT or ? WCT** try **adenosine**

if no response then:
procainamide or **amiodarone** or **sotalol** or **lidocaine** & prepare for **synch cardioversion**

irregular — **AF w/ aber.** Control rate w/ **diltiazem** or **metoprolol**

AF + WPW **amio**, proc, or ibutilide *avoid adeno, dig, CCB, βB*

PMVT (nl QT) *treat ischemia* **amio** or lidocaine & prepare for **defibrillation**

Torsades (↑ QT) *correct lytes & other precip.* **Mg** 2 g IV *overdrive pacing* or **isoproterenol**

CARDIOVERSION

Ancillary equipment
O₂ sat monitor
suction, IV line
intubation equipment

Premedicate
call anesthesia service
midazolam 1–5 mg
fentanyl 100–300 mcg

Synch cardioversion
50–200 J biphasic
100–200 J monophasic

MEDICATIONS

adenosine 6 mg *rapid* IVP then 20-mL NS bolus, 12 mg IVP q2min × 1 if needed
amiodarone 150 mg IV over 10 min
diltiazem 15–20 mg IV over 2 min, 20–25 mg 15' later prn, 5–15 mg/h
ibutilide 1 mg IV over 10 min, repeat × 1 if needed
lidocaine 1.0–1.5 mg/kg IVP, repeat in 5–10 min
metoprolol 5 mg IV q5min × 3
procainamide 17 mg/kg IV at 50 mg/min (avoid if EF ↓)
sotalol 100 mg IV over 5 min
verapamil 2.5–5 mg IV over 2 min, 5–10 mg 15–30 min later prn

(Adapted from ACLS 2010 Guidelines, *Circ* 2010;122(Suppl 3):S729)

Figure ACLS-2 ACLS Bradycardia Algorithm

BRADYCARDIA w/ Pulse (HR <50 & inadequate for clinical condition)

Airway, IV Access, O₂, monitor BP & rhythm, 12-lead ECG

(eg, hypotension, Δ MS, s/s shock, chest pain, heart failure)

Unstable? — No → **Observe**

Yes

if Type II 2° AVB or 3° AVB proceed to pacing ASAP

atropine 0.5 mg IV q3–5min, max 3 mg

transcutaneous pacing, or **dopamine** 2–10 mcg/kg/min, or **epinephrine** 2–10 mcg/min, or **isoproterenol** 2–10 mcg/min

while awaiting pacer or if pacer ineffective

transvenous pacing

(Adapted from ACLS 2010 Guidelines, *Circ* 2010;122(Suppl 3):S729)

ACLS-2

PULSELESS ARREST

1. CPR
- **C**ompressions
  - **Push hard (≥2 inches) & fast (≥100/min)**
  - Minimize interruptions; rotate compressor q2min
- **A**irway: open airway (eg, head tilt-chin lift)
- **B**reathing: ⊕ pressure ventilation; 2 breaths q 30 compressions
  - Bag-mask acceptable; supplemental O_2

Attach monitor/defibrillator ASAP

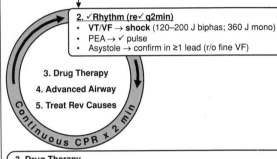

2. ✓Rhythm (re✓ q2min)
- **VT/VF → shock** (120–200 J biphas; 360 J mono)
- PEA → ✓ pulse
- Asystole → confirm in ≥1 lead (r/o fine VF)

3. Drug Therapy
4. Advanced Airway
5. Treat Rev Causes

Continuous CPR x 2 min

3. Drug Therapy
- Establish IV/IO access *(do not interrupt CPR)*
- <u>Vasopressor</u>: **epinephrine 1 mg IV q3–5min** (or 2 mg via ETT)
  - vasopressin 40 U can replace 1st or 2nd epi dose
- <u>Antiarrhythmic</u>: **amio 300 mg IVB** ± 150 mg IVB 3–5 min later
  - lidocaine 1–1.5 mg/kg IVB (~100 mg) then
    0.5–0.75 mg/kg (~50 mg) q5–10min, max 3 mg/kg
  - magnesium 1–2 g IV for TdP

4. Consider Advanced Airway
- Endotracheal intubation or supraglottic advanced airway
- Clinical assessment: bilat. chest expansion & breath sounds
- Device to ✓ tube placement
  - Continuous waveform capnography (~100% Se & Sp)
  - Colorimetric exhaled CO_2 detection (≈ clinical assess.); false neg w/ ineffective CPR, PE, pulm edema, etc.
- 8–10 breaths per min w/ continuous compressions

5. Treat Reversible Causes
- Hypovolemia: volume
- Hypoxia: oxygenate
- H^+ ions (acidosis): $NaHCO_3$
- Hypo/hyper K: KCl/Ca et al.
- Hypothermia: warm
- Tension PTX: needle decomp.
- Tamponade: pericardiocent.
- Toxins: med-specific
- Thromb. (PE): lysis, thrombect.
- Thromb. (ACS): PCI or lysis

(Adapted from ACLS 2010 Guidelines, *Circ* 2010;122(Suppl 3):S729)